CASE STUDIES
IN APHASIA
REHABILITATION

To Jon Eisenson—
for his long-standing contributions
to the clinical management of aphasic persons.

Cover portrait of Jon Eisenson by John Wilson of Austin, Texas.

FOR CLINICIANS BY CLINICIANS
Harris Winitz, Series Editor

This book, CASE STUDIES IN APHASIA REHABILITATION, is the third volume in the *For Clinicians by Clinicians* series of texts on the diagnosis and clinical management of speech, language, and voice disorders. Each text provides a contemporary perspective of one major disorder or clinical area, and is designed for use in clinical methodology courses and continuing education programs. Authors have been selected who represent a broad spectrum of clinical interests and theoretical positions, but who hold the common belief that their viewpoints, experiences, and successes should be shared in order to provide a forum *For Clinicians by Clinicians.*

Already published in this series is TREATING LANGUAGE DISORDERS and TREATING ARTICULATION DISORDERS. Other volumes are planned on cerebral palsy, cleft palate, aphasia, apraxia, dysarthria, voice, and stuttering.

CASE STUDIES IN APHASIA REHABILITATION

For Clinicians by Clinicians

Edited by
Robert C. Marshall

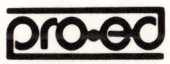

5341 Industrial Oaks Boulevard
Austin, Texas 78735

Copyright © 1986 by PRO-ED, Inc.

All rights reserved. No part of this book
may be reproduced in any form or by any means
without the prior written permission of the publisher.

Printed in the United States of America.

Library of Congress Cataloging in Publication Data

Main entry under title:

Case studies in aphasia rehabilitation.

  (For clinicians by clinicians)
  Includes bibliographies and index.
  1. Aphasics—Rehabilitation—Case studies. 2. Speech therapy—
Case studies. I. Marshall, Robert C., 1938–   . II. Series. [DNLM:
1. Aphasia—rehabilitation—case studies. WL 340.5 C337]
RC425.C38   1986   616.85′5206   85-30127
ISBN 0-89079-109-0

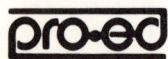

5341 Industrial Oaks Boulevard
Austin, Texas 78735

10 9 8 7 6 5 4 3 2 1   86 87 88 89 90 91

Contents

Contributors vii

Preface ix

CHAPTER 1
Rationale and Overview 1
    Robert C. Marshall

CHAPTER 2
The Patient After the Fall 19
    Deanie Vogel

CHAPTER 3
Beyond Our Usual Treatment Goals: Treatment of
a High Level Aphasic Person 31
    Marie T. Rau

CHAPTER 4
A Spouse's Role in Rehabilitation 45
    Elizabeth J. Webster

CHAPTER 5
Response to Treatment: A Case of Chronic Aphasia 59
    Robert T. Wertz

CHAPTER 6
Aphasia Treatment: Intensive and Residential 75
    Ann A. VanDemark

CHAPTER 7
Maximum Recovery: By What Definition? 89
    Sara B. Sanders

CHAPTER 8
Treatment of a Severely Aphasic Person 105
    Michael Collins

CHAPTER 9
Aphasia and Severe Apraxia of Speech:
Charting the Treatment Course 119
James L. Aten

CHAPTER 10
Evolution of Communication in a Traumatically Head
Injured Patient with Aphasia 133
Reg L. Warren

CHAPTER 11
The Center for Independent Living: A Case Study 151
Cheri L. Florance and William F. Conway

CHAPTER 12
A Social Communication Approach to Treatment
of Aphasia in an Institutional Setting 167
Rosemary Lubinski

CHAPTER 13
A Cognitive Approach to the Treatment
of Aphasia 183
Roberta Chapey

CHAPTER 14
A Case for Flexibility 197
Robert C. Marshall

CHAPTER 15
Multiple Problems and Their Effect on Speech
and Language Treatment 215
Thomas E. Prescott

CHAPTER 16
Systematic Programming of Verbal Elaboration Skills
in Chronic Broca's Aphasia 225
Kevin P. Kearns

CHAPTER 17
Computers and Caring 245
Russell H. Mills and Pamela C. Hoffer

INDEX 267

Contributors

James L. Aten, PhD
Chief, Audiology and Speech
  Pathology
Veterans Administration
  Medical Center
Long Beach, California 90822
Associate Clinical Professor,
  ENT/Head-Neck Surgery
University of California
Irvine, California

Michael J. Collins, PhD
Staff Speech Pathologist
Veterans Administration
  Medical Center
2500 Overlook Terrace
Madison, Wisconsin 53705

Roberta Chapey, EdD
Professor
Department of Speech
Brooklyn College of the
  City University of New
  York
Brooklyn, New York 11210

William F. Conway, MD
Co-Director, Center for
  Independent Living
St. Anthony Hospital
Columbus, Ohio 43203

Cheri L. Florence, PhD
Co-Director, Center for
  Independent Living
St. Anthony Hospital
Columbus, Ohio 43203

Pamela C. Hoffer, PhD
Consultant in Speech
  Pathology
Audiology and Speech
  Pathology Service
Veterans Administration
  Medical Center
Ann Arbor, Michigan 48105
Private Practice in Speech
  Pathology
Ann Arbor, Michigan

Kevin P. Kearns, PhD
Supervisor, Speech
  Pathology Section
Audiology and Speech
  Pathology Service
Veterans Administration
  Medical Center
New Orleans, Louisiana
  70146

Rosemary Lubinski, EdD
Associate Professor
Department of
  Communication Disorders
  and Science
State University of New York
  at Buffalo
Amherst, New York 14226

Robert C. Marshall, PhD
Chief, Audiology and Speech
  Pathology
Veterans Administration
  Medical Center
Portland, Oregon 97207
Assistant Professor
Department of Neurology
Oregon Health Sciences
  University
Portland, Oregon 97201

Russell H. Mills, PhD
Senior Staff Member
Audiology and Speech
  Pathology Service
Veterans Administration
  Medical Center
Ann Arbor, Michigan 48106
Director, Brain Link Software
Ann Arbor, Michigan

Thomas E. Prescott, PhD
Chief, Audiology and Speech
  Pathology Service
Veterans Administration
  Medical Center
Denver, Colorado 80220

Marie T. Rau, PhD
Chief, Speech Pathology
  Section
Audiology and Speech
  Pathology Service
Veterans Administration
  Medical Center
Portland, Oregon 97207

Sara B. Sanders, PhD
Chief, Speech Pathology
  Section
Audiology and Speech
  Pathology Service
Veterans Administration
  Medical Center
Assistant Clinical Professor
Department of
  Otolaryngology
University of Tennessee
  Center for Health Sciences
Memphis, Tennessee 38104

Ann A. VanDemark, PhD
Assistant Professor and
  Assistant Dean for
  Research
Speech and Hearing Science
University of Michigan
Ann Arbor, Michigan 48109

Deanie Vogel, PhD
Staff Speech Pathologist
Audiology and Speech
  Pathology Service
Veterans Administration
  Medical Center
Adjunct Assistant Professor
Department of Physical
  Medicine and
  Rehabilitation Health
Universtiy of Texas Health
  Science Center
San Antonio, Texas 78284

Reg L. Warren, PhD
Director, Center for
  Communication Disorders
Braintree Hospital
Braintree, Massachusetts
  02184

Elizabeth J. Webster, PhD
Professor, Department of
  Audiology and Speech
  Pathology
Memphis State University
Memphis, Tennessee 38105

Robert T. Wertz, PhD
Chief, Audiology and Speech
  Pathology
Veterans Administration
  Medical Center
Martinez, California 94553
Adjunct Associate Professor
Department of Neurology
University of California,
  Davis Medical School
Davis, California 95616

Preface

For fifteen years clinical aphasiologists have met annually throughout the United States at the Clinical Aphasiology Conference (CAC). This meeting is dedicated to the clinical management of persons with aphasia. At the CAC participants present and discuss clinical, experimental, and theoretical papers dealing with treatment processes, assessment methods, brain-behavior relationships, and other topics. However, it is in the informal interactions and discussions that occur between sessions that these clinicians talk enthusiastically about the rehabilitation of particular aphasic persons, and share their successes, failures, frustrations, and aspirations. The spirit of these interactions and the commitment of clinicans devoted to the rehabilitation of aphasic individuals have stimulated the publication of this text.

This book, the third in the *For Clinicians by Clinicians* series, contains an introductory chapter and a series of 17 case studies. Each case was actually treated by the clinician submitting the report. The names of the aphasic clients are fictitious, but what was involved in their management is factual. The cases are as varied as individual snowflakes. They have different diagnoses, prognoses, symptoms, strengths, and weaknesses. They began treatment at different times, in variable states of readiness, and with different needs.

The clinicians who so generously contributed to this textbook saw their clients in various settings: the home, hospitals, university clinics, nursing homes, and residential programs. Their methods, backgrounds, experiences, and philosophies vary. Still, they share two characteristics: (a) a commitment to the clinical management of persons with aphasia and (b) a knowledge of the "essence" of aphasia treatment.

This book is intended to illustrate that accountable and efficacious aphasia treatment results from the clinician's knowledge of the basic disorders, command of an array of clinical techniques, the ability to develop long- and short-range goals and use data from client responses to document treatment effectiveness, and the experience to make sound, independent professional judgments. Each report illustrates clearly that clinical aphasiology is both a science and an art, and that language therapy is a challenging undertaking for both clinician and patient—one that requires both creativity and perseverance.

This volume can be used by both graduate and undergraduate students in speech-language pathology as primary or supplemental reading in aphasia and other courses. Practicing aphasia clinicians will find the book invaluable in designing treatment, providing patient family counseling, and in educating other professionals, particularly physicians, as to what is involved in aphasia treatment. Professionals in fields such as neuropsychology, linguistics, and occupational and physical therapy will also find the material helpful and provocative. Finally, it is anticipated that this text will provide an impetus for aphasia clinicians to publish more case studies of aphasia rehabilitation, and that these efforts will benefit the person who counts most, the aphasic patient.

For me, the publishing of a book dedicated to the assessment, treatment, and recovery of individuals with aphasia marks the completion of a 15-year dream. I could not have accomplished this task without the support and assistance of many people. My research associate and colleague, Sandy Neuburger, has listened to me complain, and shared triumphs and setbacks for three years. For her help, unwavering support, and attention to details for which I had little time, I shall be eternally grateful. A special thank you goes to Helen Hall, my reliable, good-humored, word processor typist, who helped me complete the task around the birth of her son Adam. Motivation and support has also been abundant from the Veterans Administration, coworkers, colleagues, and friends. Finally, I would like to acknowledge Harris Winitz, editor of the *For Clinicians by Clinicians* series, for supporting the introduction of a unique text such as *Case Studies in Aphasia Rehabilitation*.

CHAPTER 1
Rationale and Overview
Robert C. Marshall

A CASE STUDY APPROACH

Several group studies indicate that speech and language rehabilitation enhances recovery from aphasia (Aten, Caligiuri, & Holland, 1982; Basso, Capitani, & Vignolo, 1979; Broida, 1977; Hagen, 1973; Holland, 1980; Marshall, Tompkins, & Phillips, 1982; Shewan & Kertesz, 1984; Wertz et al., 1981). There are also many case reports of aphasia in the neurobehavioral literature describing unusual and infrequently occurring deficits such as "alexia without agraphia" and "pure word deafness." Group studies, however, do not reveal what happened to the individual. And while reports of unusual cases provide insights as to how injury to a particular area of the brain affects speech and language, they give little information about recovery and treatment. The point of view adopted for this textbook is that an accurate picture of what occurs in language rehabilitation can come only through a careful accounting of the individual's treatment course and outcome.

Rationale

This book contains a series of treatment chronicles of patients who were treated by the clinician submitting the report. This case presentation format constitutes a departure from the manner in which aphasia and its treatment are usually presented in textbooks. Traditionally, textbooks present material in major content areas: definitions, neurological bases, testing, diagnosis, prognosis, and treatment. While this organized approach is useful in studying the disorder "aphasia," an aphasic person is not sectionable. The orientation of this textbook is therefore "wholistic" and illustrates that in clinical practice, testing, diagnosis, prognosis, and treatment are continuous, interrelated processes that start when the patient comes in the door and end when he is dismissed from treatment.

While there are many excellent aphasia textbooks available (Chapey) 1981a; Darley, 1982; Davis, 1983), none reflect what is actually involved in the management of specific patients. Sections devoted to treatment describe techniques such as Melodic Intonation Therapy (MIT)

(Sparks, 1981); Visual Action Therapy (VAT) (Helm-Estabrooks, Fitzpatrick & Barresi, 1983); and Promoting Aphasics' Communicative Effectiveness (PACE) (Davis & Wilcox, 1981). Techniques are certainly important since they help our patients communicate more effectively, but they are not "cures" for aphasia. Aphasia treatment and the practice of clinical aphasiology involve much more than knowing and applying a technique. The decisions governing the conduct of treatment are more complex.

Clinician-Client Relationship

The aim of this textbook is to capture the "essence" of what aphasia treatment is, and what it is that experienced clinical aphasiologists do to help their patients communicate optimally. Eisenson (1964) has defined language treatment as "the establishment of any relationship between a patient and a clinician in which there is recognition and understanding that improvement of communication is the purpose and goal." This textbook is intended to foster an understanding of the commitments in this relationship and of the values of aphasia treatment.

The Aphasic Person. Aphasia is a language deficit resulting from brain injury that affects the individual's ability to process symbolic information in all input (auditory, visual, tactile) and output (speaking, writing, gesturing) modalities. Brookshire (1978) has argued strongly that the word "aphasic" should be used only as an adjective. He suggests that the use of the term as a noun contributes to the depersonalization of the persons with whom aphasia clinicians work, and that it affects our attitudes toward them. This feeling is reflected in this book by the contributing clinicians who have learned to know their patients as people first, and language-disordered clients second.

A related issue concerns the use of first names by contributing clinicians to refer to their clients. As the editor, I feel that the readability of the textbook would be seriously compromised by referring to aphasic person as Mr., Mrs., or Ms. Furthermore, in the course of months or years of treatment, aphasic clinicians establish relationships with their clients on a first name basis. For these reasons I have allowed the contributors to this book to refer to their clients in the manner that is most comfortable to them.

The Aphasia Clinician. Since Paul Broca localized articulated speech in the third frontal convolution of the left frontal lobe in 1861, much has been written about aphasia. Perspectives on the disorder have been provided from many disciplines: neurology, cognitive psychology, linguistics, neuropsychology, and speech-language pathology. Research on aphasia has been abundant and the disorder has been discussed, debated, and described from many points of view.

In spite of what is known about aphasia and its the impact on the individual, the family, the environment, and the work place, what should be done to manage it is incompletely understood. For answers to these complex issues, it seems logical to turn to professionals who spend most of their time interacting and communicating with aphasic persons and their families—the aphasia clinicians themselves.

One does not become an aphasia clinician overnight. To become an aphasia clinician, one must see many aphasic patients over a prolonged period of time. This accomplishment demands study, observation, and thought. While it is possible to learn about aphasia in the classroom, from reading the literature and observing in the laboratory, it is impossible to learn much about aphasic people without spending a significant time in what Jay Rosenbek (1984) has called "the clinical trenches."

The clinicians who have contributed to this book have put in their time on the front lines. Their careers reflect a unique blending of clinical practice, research, and patient advocacy. They have chosen to share what they have learned with a particular aphasic person with those who read this book.

Organization

In this chapter, we will detail major points in each of the case studies that follow. The case studies themselves are grouped in six major themes. Chapters in part I by Deanie Vogel, Marie T. Rau, and Elizabeth J. Webster highlight the importance of counseling for the aphasic client and the family. Part II contains a set of papers by Robert T. Wertz, Ann A. VanDemark, and Sara B. Sanders on treatment of chronic aphasia.

In part III Michael J. Collins, James L. Aten, and Reg L. Warren describe methods employed and treatment results obtained with three clients suffering severe verbal expressive deficits. Cheri L. Florance and William F. Conway, and Rosemary Lubinski, in part IV, provide insights on the role of significant others in aphasia treatment in two settings, a center for independent living and a nursing home.

Part V underscores the multifaceted nature of aphasia treatment and the need for clinician flexibility. Roberta Chapey describes a cognitively based treatment approach employed with a high level aphasic man. Robert C. Marshall and Thomas E. Prescott describe the management of two aphasic men who suffered multiple setbacks in the course of their recovery (second strokes, illness) necessitating the refocusing of their treatment. Part VI contains two chapters. In the first Kevin P. Kearns reports how a multiple baseline single subject design treatment method was used to promote spontaneous verbal elaboration skills in a

Broca's aphasic client. In addition, he illustrates how data from a clinical trial may be used to measure treatment effects that may escape recognition on standardized tests. In the final chapter, Russell H. Mills and Pamela C. Hoffer describe how microcomputers were used in the management of two clients. The first was a young aphasic man whose treatment involved application of microcomputer programs to provide "massed practice." The second was a young head injured client who was assisted in his activities of daily living by a microcomputer used to compensate for some of his cognitive deficits.

Each case study is prefaced by a brief introductory statement that focuses the chapter and a series of study questions that challenge the reader's understanding of the clinical material presented.

Theoretical Bases

This textbook differs from some others in that it does not provide a theoretical basis for aphasia therapy. Instead, it focuses on what was done in the assessment, treatment, decision to terminate treatment, and follow-up of 17 patients.

Nevertheless, some chapters do provide theoretical perspectives on salient issues. Wertz (chapter 5), for example, summarizes the prevailing opinions on the advisability of treating chronic aphasia. Warren (chapter 10) provides theoretical insights on the facilitating effects of an augmentative communication system for a patient whose speech suddenly returned at 4½ years post onset. Kearns (chapter 16) offers insights on the use of single subject experimental designs in determining the effects of aphasia treatment. And Chapey (chapter 13) reviews some of the assumptions underlying a cognitively based approach to language treatment. While other chapters provide some theoretical background, the primary orientation of each is clinical and practical.

COUNSELING AND TREATMENT

The papers in part I by Vogel, Rau, and Webster are examples of the role aphasia clinicians play in counseling aphasic persons and their families. They provide insights on what it is like to be an aphasic person and/or a member of an aphasic person's family. Each author offers some indication of the patient's fears (e.g., uncontrolled emotional lability), concerns (e.g., returning to work), and problems (e.g., driving) that arise in treatment. From the clinician's handling of these issues and the counseling they provided to deal with them, the reader can appreciate the effects aphasia has not only on the patient, but also on the family.

"Relative" Impact of Aphasia

Vogel and Rau describe the speech and language rehabilitation of two professional men, one a dentist, the other a college instructor. While each patient quickly recovered "functional communication," the lives of each were devastated by mild communication deficits that interfered with returning to work. These two patients' reactions to deficits that would be perceived by most as "minor" indicate that the impact of aphasia is relative to the person's dependence on and need to use language in his or her life.

Vogel's client refused to accept anything short of a total recovery. He describes what it is like to be aphasic in terms of his comprehension and word retrieval problems, and he vents his reactions toward others whom he perceived as "not listening" or "talking down to him." He also provides us with an insider's view on what the clinician can do to help: be patient, facilitate responses, and "treat me as a peer with dignity."

The college instructor treated by Rau regained functional communication skills rapidly following a stroke. His speech and writing, however, were not so proficient that he could return to his profession; he became overly critical of his errors and hypersensitive to the reactions of others. Through intensive counseling and developing strategies to optimize communication, Rau assisted the client and his wife in reducing his self-deprecating behaviors.

High Level Clients

Another important point in Rau's and Vogel's chapters concerns the opportunity and the time to treat mildly aphasic clients. In some clinics, the fact that both patients had become functional communicators before entering treatment may have precluded their receiving treatment. But, as Rau's title suggests. It is important to work "beyond our usual treatment goals." She carefully prepared her client for return to teaching. When he did return to the classroom, she provided long-term follow-up, feedback, and critiques of his lessons to ease his transition into the working world. Vogel employed a step-by-step desensitization process with her client in which he had to speak in situations of increasing difficulty to prepare him for communication on the job.

The Patient's Judgment

Schuell, Jenkins, and Jiminez-Pabon (1964) suggested that when the aphasic patient thinks he can return to work, the clinician should trust this judgment rather than the results of standardized tests. This axiom is applicable in both the Rau and Vogel cases. Both clients returned to work but the clinicians who provided the treatment had reservations as to whether working on a full-time basis, at prior levels of performance, would be possible. It was necessary for both Rau and Vogel to step back and let their clients try. This tactic illustrates the importance of enabling patients to experience their own failures and frustrations before setting limits. Once these limits have been established it is important for clinicians to "be there" to assist and counsel clients in setting realistic limits.

Family Counseling

The final paper in part I (chapter 4) is a unique account of a severely aphasic man. I use the term "unique" without reservation because the author, Betty Webster, has vividly described her client's treatment through changes in the perceptions and attitudes of his wife. This account spans a two-year period during which the wife participated in a spouses' counseling group and her aphasic husband received speech and language therapy at the Memphis State University Speech and Hearing Clinic. This report is written in a distinctly personalized style. Webster's use of quotations from counseling sessions, spouse-client interactions, and clinician-spouse exchanges depicts clearly problems that come up when a member of a family suffers from aphasia: independence, questions of driving, and the need to accept a less than perfect communication system.

Webster describes how a combination of client treatment and counseling of the the spouse enabled each to learn to cope with and adjust to persistent and severe aphasic deficits. The chapter illustrates the need to include the "significant others" in the treatment process, and how behaviors and attitudes of these persons shape the patient's treatment course.

TREATMENT OF CHRONIC APHASIA

Rising health care costs have raised concerns about when aphasia treatment should begin, how often it should be provided, and how long it should continue. Improvements in the medical management of stroke have increased the survival rate; thus, we will probably see an increase in the numbers of chronic aphasic clients. Many could benefit from more treatment but most cannot get it because (a) there is no way to pay for it and/or (b) busy clinicians are occupied with providing services to acute patients for whom insurance coverage is available.

Group studies illustrate that chronic patients who receive treatment long after spontaneous recovery has ended and "optimum" treatment windows have closed make significant progress in treatment (Broida, 1977; Aten, Caligiuri, & Holland, 1982; Smith, 1972). Perhaps our best evidence that aphasia treatment "works" comes from cases who make marked progress when their treatment is provided in the chronic state. The three cases of part II from Wertz, VanDemark, and Sanders provide this kind of documentation.

Should We Treat Chronic Aphasia?

Wertz's chapter, "Response to Treatment: A Case of Chronic Aphasia," summarizes what is known about the advisability of treating chronic cases—basically, "not much." Although early treatment has been stressed (Basso et al., 1979; Marshall et al., 1982; Wertz et al., 1981), Wertz's client and the other two cases reported in part II made significant progress when treated in the chronic state. It seems additional information is needed before making up our minds.

Wertz's report documents the effects of speech and language treatment with a man who lived with his aphasic deficits for seven years before re-entering treatment. Not only did the man make progress in 2½ years of additional treatment, but he decided he wanted to return to work and "drop off" the welfare roles. He improved in treatment but he eventually leveled off in his performance on formal tests such as the *Porch Index of Communicative Ability* (PICA). (Porch, 1971). His clinician did, however, succeed in getting him back to work. This necessitated some special effort and it suggests yet another role for the clinical aphasiologist, that of patient advocate.

At three years postonset, VanDemark's patient was enrolled for the first of four 10-week sessions in the Residential Aphasia Clinic (RAC) at the University of Michigan. In the RAC he received intensive treatment (four to six hours daily). Early RAC treatment focused on improving speech and language skills on basic levels, but his final 10-week session in the RAC was intended to promote language skills needed if and when he returned to his former occupation as a social worker. In this chapter, VanDemark illustrates the value of using different treatment strategies at different points in recovery.

Intensity. Little is known about how frequently aphasic clients should be seen for treatment. This decision is often dictated by factors other than clinician judgment (e.g., money, geography, time) and certainly not by any available data. VanDemark points out in the treatment of her client that when aphasia is chronic, intensive treatment may be warranted. In her report, she is careful to document progress made by the client in each RAC session through careful objective testing in reading, listening, and with various standardized language measures such as the PICA and *Boston Diagnostic Aphasia Exam*

(BDAE), (Goodglass & Kaplan, 1972). Results show that the client progressed when he had treatment, and regressed or did not change when he was not in treatment.

Both the Wertz and VanDemark cases provide strong evidence that treatment of chronic aphasia can be beneficial, particularly when it fosters increased independence and a possible return to gainful employment.

Termination of Treatment

The final paper in part II by Sanders addresses the issue of termination of treatment. She describes the treatment course of a young and relatively chronic aphasic man, who progressed in his initial stint of individual therapy, "plateaued" on the PICA, and was dismissed from individual therapy. Eventually, he asked to be re-enrolled in treatment to work on goals that were very meaningful to him. These included (a) reducing response latencies and (b) communicating in longer, more complex sentences. Sanders' paper, "Maximum Recovery: By What Definition," is appropriately titled. After the client's PICA performance suggested that he was not changing, he made substantial gains upon re-enrollment in treatment designed to meet his needs. These gains were reflected in his improved verbal communication and on the PICA as well.

The Patient's Goal. Sanders' report also supports the need to treat chronic aphasic patients and pointedly illustrates how we may obtain better results with some clients when we let them set their own goals. This aspect of treatment can be particularly important when the goals in question are of vital concern to the patient. Finally, as Sanders points out in her case report, we need to remember that standardized tests do not always reflect the results of our treatment. We need to look for other ways to measure change.

MANAGEMENT OF SEVERE VERBAL COMMUNICATION DEFICITS

In most of the cases presented in this textbook, the primary focus in treatment was to improve verbal communication. In planning treatment for the client with a severe verbal communication deficit, the clinical aphasiologist must determine whether to shore up the damaged verbal system, bypass it entirely, or develop compensatory forms of communication. Making this decision is difficult because it is clear that our patients want to talk, that their families want them to talk, and that society judges therapeutic success by whether or not they are able to talk. For the three cases in this section by Collins, Aten, and

Warren the prognosis for developing functional verbal communication was questionable. Therefore a decision had to be made whether to push for verbal communication or promote the use of compensatory techniques.

Global Aphasia

In chapter 8, Collins describes his treatment of a globally aphasic man, who in the early phases of treatment actually refused to participate in treatment or formal testing. Patience and perseverance while providing the client with some successes led to establishing sufficient rapport for the patient to enter treatment willingly. When this occurred, however, he refused anything that did not promise speech. Collins describes methods that encouraged the patient to use a total communication approach involving a combination of gesturing, writing, drawing, and speech.

Severe Apraxia

In chapter 9, Aten documents the treatment of an aphasic man whose language deficits were markedly compounded by a severe oral and verbal apraxia that rendered him speechless. Treatment was provided to re-establish voluntary control of speech at basic levels: initiation of phonation, producing continuant sounds, and automatic speech. Unfortunately, systematic treatment of the patient's deficits at these basic levels did not lead to improved verbal communication.

One of the most important points from Aten's paper is that what we "hope" for in treatment and what the patient can achieve may be incompatible. Aten's use of treatment data to support whether or not continuancy training for rebuilding speech is noteworthy. It shows the value of basing treatment results on data rather than wishes. It also raises the question of when to try an augmentative communicative approach, an issue Warren covers in the third paper in this set.

Mutism

In chapter 10, Warren describes the 9-year treatment course of a young head-injured patient with aphasia. The client was almost speechless for 4¼ years. During this time he learned to use a total communication approach involving gesturing, a speech notebook, writing, and a few words. This approach was not usable in a work setting, so the patient was taught to use an augmentative device (Handi-Voice) that allowed him to communicate using synthesized speech. At 4½ years postonset the patient's speech returned suddenly. Within a few weeks, his verbal output resembled that of a patient with Broca's aphasia. Continued treatment emphasized the combined use of the speech synthesizer and verbal communication. Eventually, the client discarded the speech synthesizer and relied solely on verbal communication. He returned to work. In this paper, Warren offers some interesting observations on the facilitating effects of augmentative devices.

The Importance of Speech

The cases presented by Collins, Aten, and Warren highlight the importance of verbal communication to our aphasic patients. But, they also raise questions about the value of pursuing verbal communication with *all* clients. Collins' patient accepted and learned to use a total communication approach, but he continued to strive to perfect this communication system. Aten's client failed to regain usable verbal communication but was observed to generate well-articulated utterances in relaxed nonthreatening situations. Warren's case was silent for 4¼ years; then the use of an augmentative device seemed to facilitate the return of speech.

Until more information is available, clinical aphasiologists will have to grapple with the decision to pursue verbal communication or to promote the use of compensatory efforts. It is possible that we may deprive our patients of the opportunity to communicate by not introducing total communication systems or augmentative devices first. Dwelling on talking when this endeavor is destined to fail may create an attitude of failure. While early introduction of compensatory systems may be helpful, the information presented here suggests that "the hope for speech dies hard," and it is not the clinician's job to destroy this hope. It is the clinician's job to promote communication and to capitalize on those "islands" of strength that emerge and offer a promise for further verbalization.

SIGNIFICANT OTHERS AND TREATMENT

The aphasic client spends a fraction of the day in speech and language therapy. Some communicate very well in the relaxed atmosphere of the clinic with the support of the aphasia clinician, but fall to pieces under the communicative pressures of the real world. It is unrealistic to assume that the patient's performance in treatment will generalize automatically to situations outside the clinic. Generalization needs to be planned for, and perhaps one means of accomplishing this is to involve the patient's significant other(s) in the treatment process itself.

Many of the chapters in this book indicate the necessity of including the patient's significant others in treatment, but Florance and Conway, in chapter 11, and Lubinski, in chapter 12, suggest this is essential.

Center for Independent Living

Florance and Conway co-direct a model program for the medical management and rehabilitation of the elderly individual in Columbus, Ohio. This program, the Center for Independent Living (CIL), is designed to promote the autonomy and independence of its clients. The CIL reflects a strong interdisciplinary orientation where people from the fields of medicine, speech-language pathology, occupational therapy, psychology, and other disciplines function as a team to make recommendations and devise treatment strategies to return the patient to independent living status.

Evaluation. In the CIL, the patient undergoes a thorough evaluation by representatives of each discipline. The focus of this evaluation differs from rehabilitation efforts that divide the patient into parts, and each discipline, including speech pathology, concentrates solely on its area of expertise. The CIL assessments analyze the patient's coping and compliance mechanisms, assess ADL skills in simulated settings such as a bank, and review driving and transportation needs. Evaluation of the patient's communication efficiency is based on how well the client performs in the environment with members of the family, rather than the interpretation of the results of standardized tests.

Reports from the CIL for Florance and Conway's patient have been included in some detail. By reading these reports carefully, the reader will appreciate that appropriate evaluation generates appropriate recommendations and treatment plans. The CIL is geared toward short-term treatment and the rapid transfer of skills learned in the clinic to outside situations. This process begins almost immediately upon the patient's admission to the program. Success is heavily dependent on the assistance of significant others and the education of these persons by the speech-language pathologist or the most appropriate professional.

Role of Speech, Language and Cognition. In the CIL, communication and cognitive abilities are integral aspects of the total program, not peripheral skills to be worked on if the patient has a communication problem such as aphasia. Florance and Conway's patient entered the CIL depressed, noncommunicative, and was waiting for a nursing home bed. Within a few weeks and only 15 hours of treatment, she regained her independent living status and resumed many of her former recreational pursuits.

Institutionalized Aphasic Clients

In chapter 12, Lubinski describes the types of aphasic clients typically residing in nursing homes. She points out that these individuals present severe speech, language, and cognitive deficits of a long-standing duration that are compounded by the effects of aging and institutionalization. Lubinski suggests that changes that occur in traditional speech and language therapy with nursing home clients are not likely to generalize to the patient's environment. She emphasizes that, without appropriate intervention, these clients return to an environment where there are few opportunities to communicate.

In her treatment of a severely aphasic woman, Lubinski details strategies for breaking down physical and psychological barriers in a nursing home that prevent aphasic clients from using the communicative skills they possess. Her social communication approach was designed to involve significant others in treatment and to "shift the burden of communicative responsibility" from the profoundly impaired client and the clinician to significant others who care for the client (e.g., nurse, aide, physical therapist).

Role Changes. Lubinski found it necessary to move out of the treatment room and see her client on the ward where significant others would see what was going on. By divesting herself of "clinical trappings" and permitting others to see her interacting with the patient, she presented the client as a potential communicator, encouraged caregivers to talk to her, and reinforced them for their efforts.

It is refreshing that Lubinski does not minimize the severity of her client's deficits nor those of institutionalized aphasic patients. She provides insights on some of the problems in implementing a social communication approach in a nursing home: professional image, documentation, and getting others involved. As Lubinski suggests in her chapter, we need to rethink the manner in which we provide treatment to nursing home patients.

CLINICIAN FLEXIBILITY

Aphasia treatment is not static. It is a dynamic, ever-changing process. The clinician is making continuous decisions about the direction treatment should take. Treatment goals need to be adjusted in accordance with the client's needs and abilities; the clinician may need to review what is done in treatment in relation to what is happening in the client's life. Chapters 13, 14, and 15 by Chapey, Marshall, and Prescott illustrate the variety of decisions that need to be made and the flexibility required in making them.

Language and Thought

Many believe that aphasia treatment should focus on stimulation of those thoughts and ideas underlying language (Chapey, 1981a; 1981b;

Martin, 1981; Wepman, 1972, 1976). In chapter 13, Chapey presents a cognitive approach for the treatment of aphasia. Her patient was a 68-year-old man who was so frustrated by his aphasic deficits that he avoided communication entirely. Chapey determined that the patient was able to use "words" as demonstrated by his normal performance on standardized exams; but he was impaired in use of the underlying cognitive processes supporting language.

In her treatment program, Chapey provides us with specific tasks designed to promote cognition, memory, evaluative thinking, convergent and divergent thinking, and combinations of these skills. Treatment was intended to promote flexibility in thinking, problem solving, and decision making. Treatment tasks are inherently practical. For example, Chapey had the patient detail the steps in planning a trip, discuss the pros and cons of owning a home, and summarize material from a newspaper article.

The reader will see similarities between Chapey's case and Rau's patient (chapter 2). Both were higher level aphasic clients who were frustrated by their mild deficits. Treatment with each involved conversation within the imposed structure of Wepman's content centered thought therapy (Wepman, 1972) and of PACE therapy (Davis & Wilcox, 1981). Both cases demonstrate that the impact of aphasia is relative to the person's dependence on language and that treatment needs to be provided to the higher level client.

The Road to Recovery

In chapters 14 and 15, Marshall and Prescott describe the rather complicated treatment courses of two aphasic men. Both papers illustrate that the road to recovery from aphasia takes many turns, some of them unexpected. Prescott's patient suffered two major medical setbacks in his treatment course. Marshall's patient incurred a second stroke and had to cope with major changes in his life that necessitated him resuming a leadership role in his family.

The treatment courses for both of these men reflect the many decisions that clinicians have to make in treating a given patient. These include adjusting and refocusing treatment, determining when to end treatment, and postponing treatment until the patient overcomes other deficits. Above all, each case illustrates the need to maintain a high degree of flexibility in the treatment of aphasic persons.

The reader will want to pay particular attention to the methods used by Marshall to minimize his client's word retrieval deficits. Similarly, Prescott's treatment of his client's auditory comprehension deficits and the use of a "verbing program" (Loverso, Selinger, & Prescott, 1979) to enhance the use of longer sentence construction offer practical treatment methods. Both papers provide an indication of how clinical data can be used to document treatment effects and to plan treatment.

Finally, the chapters by Marshall and Prescott highlight the commitment of the clinical aphasiologist to evaluate the results of treatment on a periodic basis. Both patients were tested monthly with the PICA. PICA data provided a measure of treatment effects and also yielded information about what was occurring with the patient. Both patients demonstrated a noticeable drop in performance on the PICA before their second strokes, further emphazing the need for periodic objective evaluation.

SCIENTIFIC INQUIRY AND TREATMENT

In summarizing a series of Clinical Aphasiology Conference papers on the use of single subject designs in aphasia treatment, Davis (1978) suggested that the medical profession is deserving of "our data and not our word." Chapter 16 by Kearns epitomizes the importance of using data from the clinic to evaluate what we "feel" occurs in aphasia treatment.

Clinical Data

Kearns states that standardized testing is necessary to document the results of aphasia treatment, but it may be insufficient as the sole means of accomplishing this. He makes a strong case for the use of data from treatment tasks as a means of measuring change. Kearns suggests (a) that treatment tasks may not be included in a standardized test battery and (b) that the time elapsing between test points may be too great to reflect what occurs in day-to-day treatment. In such cases, inappropriate treatment decisions might be the unfortunate result. Objective evaluation of treatment on a regular basis assists the clinician to determine whether treatment is helpful, and it permits adjustments in the conduct of treatment when they are needed rather than after the fact.

Treatment Designs

Kearns and others (Davis, 1978; LaPointe, 1978, 1984; Thompson & Kearns, 1981) have provided models of aphasia treatment plans that fall within subject experimental design methodologies. These designs permit the clinician to support "assumed" cause-effect relationships between treatment and behavioral change, and to assess the generalization of treated stimuli and/or tasks to untreated stimuli. The importance of planning for generalization was mentioned in the section on the role of significant others in treatment (chapter 10), and in the continuancy program described by Aten in chapter 9. However, the methods used by Kearns are more specific and allow the clinician to determine whether or not generalization has occurred.

Baseline Data. Theoretically, if the aphasic patient is not performing at a stable rate on a treatment task, improvement on that task cannot be attributed to treatment alone. Kearns details procedures for establishing baseline levels, defining acceptable responses, setting criterion performance in treatment, and determining whether treatment efforts generalize to untreated stimuli. These methods can be applied clinically to document what we do: in treatment planning, for referral sources, and for those who pay the bills.

Communication vs. Linguistic Form. Kearns' case presentation differentiates between treatment designed to promote communicative function and that intended to improve linguistic accuracy. His treatment for a chronic Broca's aphasic client was designed to promote initiation and elaboration of spontaneous responses on a picture description task. Kearns describes the clinical procedures used and contributes something novel to clinical aphasiology. This involves the use of "loose training" strategies (Stokes & Baer, 1977) in which (a) Kearns shaped and elaborated upon spontaneously produced client responses rather than targeting preselected responses and (b) the communicative success attained when the patient-initiated response was given priority over the use of a specific linguistic structure as a means of communicating.

Kearns' client made significant improvements in spontaneous speech production. This was reflected on treated stimuli. Treatment effects generalized to nontreated items with which the client was familiar. Further, improvement was noted on independent overall measures of language (e.g., PICA) as well. While the progress of the patient is important, the lessons provided from the report are equally important. They tell us that our treatment can be more scientific, accountable, and rigorous, yet remain uniquely human.

Computerized Treatment

Microcomputers are being used to perform a variety of tasks that clinicians usually perform as a part of treatment. When properly utilized, microcomputers can save the clinician time in record keeping, scoring, and analysis of data sets. One only has to compare the time it takes a clinician with the time it takes a computer to do the mathematical computations for the PICA to realize how true this is.

In chapter 17, Mills and Hoffer explain how microcomputers were used to augment clinicians' efforts in the management of two clients. The first client was severely aphasic. That portion of his treatment carried out by microcomputer followed traditional lines. The second client exhibited cognitive deficits secondary to a closed head injury. His treatment by microcomputer was nontraditional and involved the use of the word processor and other features of the system.

Traditional Microcomputer Use. By "traditional," Mills and Hoffer refer to programs in reading, auditory comprehension, math, general information, and other areas that provide the user massed practice on a task. These tasks tend to be relatively straightforward and are often tedious for the clinician to administer. Computer administration saves time for the clinician, but more importantly, it allows the patient to work at his or her own rate of speed. As a consequence, a patient may work longer, at higher success rates, and with less frustration. Feedback and reinforcement can be provided by the computer. In addition, the computer can be programmed to adjust certain parameters (e.g., speed of presentation, rate of speech) contingent on the user's response.

Nontraditional Application. With their head injured client, the authors explored some new microcomputer applications to treatment. The client's language was relatively intact. His major deficits were memory, reduced speech intelligibility secondary to spastic dysarthria, and difficulty in initiating communication. He was taught to use the word processing feature of a microcomputer system to produce written correspondence and to help him remember things to discuss with his wife. In teaching computer tasks to his four-year-old son, he was required to use a pattern of patient/child interaction that was modeled for him. He was able to use the financial management package of the system to pay bills. With the assistance of the computer, he resumed some of his former responsibilities as father and husband, and regained much of his self-esteem.

Computer or Clinician?

Mills and Hoffer suggest the microcomputer should not be considered as a replacement for the clinician. But, when appropriately utilized it can augment the clinician's efforts. They indicate that each of their clients improved with computerized treatment, but this treatment was only part of a total treatment program and was not necessarily responsible for gains in other areas. They fairly describe the possibilities and limitations of microcomputer use in speech-language pathology. From their chapter, the reader will realize that the future looks bright for the increased application of this technology in aphasia treatment and that practicing clinicians will need to learn to apply it. Or, as Minifie (1983) stated in his plea for more clinical research in speech-language pathology, "Someone else will do it for us."

ACCOUNTABILITY

A strong accountability theme surfaces in every chapter in this book. This translates to our being responsible for what we do as aphasia clinicians. Being accountable involves much more than giving the aphasic patient a PICA regularly to see if scores have gone up to prove treatment is working. Being accountable entails making decisions about when treatment should begin, end, or change directions. It involves evaluating behavioral change in terms of things that make a difference in the patient's life such as returning to work or resuming abandoned social activities.

Concerned clinicians take the time to evaluate their work frequently and to ask if what they are doing is helping the patient. From the descriptions of the treatment provided the 17 individuals in this book, the answer appears to be "yes."

REFERENCES

Aten, J., Caligiuri, M., & Holland, A. (1982). The efficacy of functional communication therapy for chronic aphasic patients. *Journal of Speech and Hearing Disorders, 47,* 93–96.

Basso, A., Capitani, E., & Vignolo, L.A. (1979). Influence of rehabilitation on language skills in aphasic patients: A controlled study. *Archives of Neurology, 36,* 190–196.

Broida, H. (1977). Language therapy effects in long term aphasia. *Archives Physical Medicine Rehabilitation, 58,* 248–253.

Brookshire, R.H. (1978). *An Introduction to aphasia.* Minneapolis: BRK Publishers.

Chapey, R. (1981a). *Language intervention strategies in adult aphasia.* Baltimore: Williams & Wilkins.

Chapey, R. (1981b). Divergent semantic intervention. In R. Chapey (Ed), *Language intervention strategies in adult aphasia.* Baltimore: Williams & Wilkins.

Darley, F.E. (1982). *Aphasia.* Philadelphia: W.B. Saunders.

Davis. A.G. (1983). *A survey of adult aphasia.* Englewood Cliffs. NJ: Prentice-Hall.

Davis, A.G. (1978). "Our data not our word." In R. Brookshire (Ed.), *Clinical Aphasiology Conference Proceedings.* Minneapolis: BRK Publishers.

Davis, A.G., & Wilcox, M.J. (1981). Incorporating parameters of natural language in aphasia treatment. In R. Chapey (Ed.), *Language intervention strategies in adult aphasia.* Baltimore: Williams & Wilkins.

Eisenson, J. (1964). Aphasia: A point of view as to the disorder and factors that determine prognosis for recovery. *International Journal of Neurology, 4,* 287–295.

Goodglass, H., & Kaplan E. (1972). *Assessment of aphasia and related disorders.* Philadelphia: Lea & Febiger.

Hagen, C. (1973). Communicative abilities in hemiplegia: Effect of speech and language therapy. *Archives of Physical Medicine Rehabilitation. 54,* 454–463.

Helm-Estabrooks, N.A., Fitzpatrick, P.M., & Barresi, B. (1983). Visual action therapy for global aphasia. *Journal of Speech and Hearing Disorders, 47*, 385-389.

Holland, A. (1980). The usefulness of treatment for aphasia: A serendipitous study. In R. Brookshire (Ed.), *Clinical Aphasiology Conference Proceedings*. Minneapolis: BRK Publishers.

LaPointe, L. (1978). Multiple baseline designs. In R. Brookshire (Ed.), *Clinical Aphasiology Conference Proceedings*. Minneapolis: BRK Publishers.

LaPointe, L. (1984). Sequential treatment of split lists: A case report. In J. Rosenbek, M. McNeil, & A. Aronson (Eds.), *Apraxia of speech*. San Diego: College Hill Press.

Loverso, F., Selinger, J., & Prescott, T.E. (1979). Application of verbing strategies to aphasia treatment. In R. Brookshire (Ed.), *Clinical Aphasiology Conference Proceedings*. Minneapolis: BRK Publishers.

Marshall, R.C., Tompkins, C.A., & Phillips, D.S. (1982). Improvement in treated aphasia: Examination of selected prognostic factors. *Folia Phoniatrica 34*, 305-315.

Martin, A.D. (1981). An examination of Wepman's thought-centered therapy. In R. Chapey (Ed.), *Language intervention strategies in adult aphasia*. Baltimore: Williams & Wilkins.

Minifie, F. (1983). *Presidential Address, American Speech-Language-Hearing Association*. Cincinnati.

Porch, B.E. (1971). *Porch Index of Communicative Ability*. Palo Alto, CA: Consulting Psychologists.

Rosenbek, J.C. (1984). Personal Communication.

Schuell, H., Jenkins, J.J., & Jiminez-Pabon, E. (1964). *Aphasia in adults*. New York: Harper & Row.

Shewan, C.M., & Kertesz, A. (1984). Effects of speech and language treatment on recovery from aphasia. *Brain and Language, 23*, 272-299.

Smith, A. (1972). *Diagnosis, intelligence, and rehabilitation of chronic aphasics: Final report*. University of Michigan, Department of Physical Medicine and Rehabilitation, Ann Arbor, MI.

Sparks, R. (1981). Melodic intonation therapy. In R. Chapey (Ed.), *Language intervention strategies in adult aphasia*. Baltimore: Williams & Wilkins.

Stokes, T.F., & Baer, D.M. (1977). An implicit technology of generalization. *Journal of Applied Behavior Analysis. 10*, 349-367.

Thompson, C.K., & Kearns, K.P. (1981). An experimental analysis of acquisition, generalization, and maintenance of naming behavior in a patient with anomia. In R. Brookshire (Ed.), *Clinical Aphasiology Conference Proceedings*. Minneapolis: BRK Publishers.

Wepman, J.M. (1972). Aphasia therapy: A new look. *Journal of Speech and Hearing Disorders, 37*, 203-214.

Wepman, J.M. (1976). Language without thought or thought without language. *ASHA, 18*, 131-136.

Wertz, R.T., Collins. M.J., Weiss, D., Kurtzke, J.F., et al. (1981). Veterans Administration cooperative study on aphasia: A comparison of individual and group treatment. *Journal of Speech and Hearing Research, 24*, 580-594.

CHAPTER 2
The Patient After the Fall
Deanie Vogel

> Vogel illustrates the importance of addressing the concerns of the "high level" mildly impaired aphasic patient. The author describes a treatment approach that assisted the patient in coping with his high performance expectations in communication and work. Most important, she provides a perspective on aphasia, the disorder, and aphasia treatment from the patient's point of view.
>
> 1. Distinguish between the approaches used in the treatment of apraxia of speech described by Rosenbek and his colleagues (1973, 1978) and those used by Vogel. How do these approaches differ?
> 2. How do the indirect treatment procedures employed by the author compare to Wepman's (1972) thought centered therapy?
> 3. Vogel describes a hierarchy of speaking situations that was used to desensitize the patient to listeners' reactions to his speech errors outside the clinic. What is the objective of this procedure?

THE FALL

Background

In the winter of 1981, Tim was 30 years old, a dentist and a major in the military. He had been assigned to duty in Germany near mountains where, while on leave, he could practice skiing, a sport he enjoyed. His wife was with him. With a satisfying marriage and a promising career, Tim was looking forward to the future.

Then, one day while skiing, Tim fell and hit the occipital area of the left side of his head. He thought it was "just another fall," and reported that he felt sort of shaken but not particularly hurt. The next day, while skiing again, he fell once more, this time hitting the left parietal area of his head. One hour later, Tim was admitted to a nearby hospital where he was observed for six days. He was discharged with a diagnosis of cerebral concussion.

Two weeks later Tim was admitted to the hospital on his military base complaining of severe head pain extending down to his jaw. By the next day the headache had worsened and he was disoriented. He could not answer questions regarding the date, year, or where he was stationed. According to the hospital records, he was unable to say the words he wanted to say, although his understanding of speech appeared to be adequate.

A CT scan showed a diffuse intracerebral hematoma with a massive left to right shift of the midline structures. A craniotomy was performed and a subdural hematoma of the left fronto-temporal area was removed.

Early Intervention

Two weeks following surgery, a speech-language pathologist administered the *Sklar Aphasia Scale* (Sklar, 1966). Tim achieved a total impairment score of 24, which, according to Sklar, indicates good prognosis for recovery. The examiner noted that Tim had difficulty following complex commands. He could name and categorize common objects, but as the length and difficulty of verbal output tasks increased, perseverative, paraphasic, and articulatory errors became more prevalent. Early speech and language therapy was designed to improve Tim's volitional production of selected functional phrases. An eight-step task continuum described by Rosenbek, Lemme, Ahern, Harris, and Wertz (1973) was followed. The final report written at the conclusion of 20 treatment sessions indicated that he was producing phrases such as "I want down" and "I am thirsty."

Tim's drive to recover his physical abilities and his annoyance with his speech errors was documented frequently in his medical records. A note written by a member of the rehabilitation team shortly before he left the military hospital indicated that he propelled himself in his wheelchair, but sometimes overextended himself dangerously. The speech-language pathologist wrote that "Major D. demonstrates much frustration with his speech and is very hard on himself when he does not produce words correctly."

Six weeks following surgery, Tim was air-evacuated to the United States and was admitted to the Rehabilitation Medicine Service of the Veterans Administration Hospital in San Antonio, Texas. The social worker's report shortly after his admission read as follows:

> Dr. D. is a very cooperative and pleasant patient. He has a very positive attitude about his rehabilitation and hopes to return to his dental profession. He has a close relationship with his wife and is very positive about the future. He does not allow his position as a medical professional to interfere with his being a patient on the unit. He respects limits and follows ward regulations. He is alert, cooperative, and very eager to maintain his independence and to return to his profession and his previous life.

The consultation request sent to speech-language pathology read: "Closed head injury; left hematoma evacuation, right hemiparesis and expressive aphasia." In April 1981, Tim became a patient in the speech-language pathology clinic.

SPEECH AND LANGUAGE EVALUATION

Tim was administered the *Boston Diagnostic Aphasia Examination* (BDAE) (Goodglass & Kaplan, 1972). His overall severity rating was 3, indicating that he could discuss everyday problems with little assistance; however, reduction of his available vocabulary made conversation about certain material difficult. On the basis of his expository speech and auditory comprehension scores, the diagnosis of aphasia, Broca's type, was determined. Tim's auditory comprehension was good; he followed complex commands appropriately and responded to complex ideational material accurately. His verbal output consisted of halting, dysfluent speech with articulatory errors involving transpositions of phonemes, repetitions of words, and a high incidence of filled pauses (e.g., "um," "ooh"). Audible groping for correct phonemes occurred frequently. Tim's description of the "Cookie Theft" picture from the BDAE appears below:

> The..um..boy..boy..is following, following, following..no..falling off the stool and um.. the s sink is over-fhlowing..um.. She is laughing at the boy. um..the..um.. She is reaching for the cookie..um..jar..ooh.

Reading comprehension was within normal limits. Oral reading revealed errors similar to those identified in conversation and picture description. Writing was intelligible; some spelling errors were present on a writing-to-dictation task, particularly in complex, multisyllabic words (e.g., "physician").

A motor speech evaluation was administered. Tim was unsuccessful in a diadochokinetic rate task requiring him to produce sequences of the monosyllables, *puh, tuh,* and *kuh.* He repeated the multisyllabic words "gingerbread," "snowman," and "television" with no difficulty; however, repeating multisyllabic words five times (e.g., "artillery") resulted in audible groping and phoneme substitutions. For example, when asked to attempt five productions of the word "impossibility," he responded with the following:

Imbossibility..um..tin.gin..ooh..im poss i bili ty..din..bin..ooh.. I can't.

Monosyllabic words in which identical phonemes occurred in the initial and final position in a word (e.g., "mom," "lull") were presented. Tim repeated most of the words with no difficulty. An exception was the word "zoos." His response consisted of audible groping followed by correct production of the word,

um..du..cu..ooh..who..no..cu..zoos.

He also had difficulty producing words having the same root, but increasing in length. For example, he repeated correctly the word "zip" but his response to "zipper" was a groping, "dip, dip, dipper" and for "zippering" he said "zipper wing." Deletions and substitutions of phonemes were noted during sentence repetition. For example, when repeating the sentence "In the summer they sell vegetables," Tim said:

In the summer they shell..um..ve-ge-bles.

Similar errors were exhibited in oral reading as illustrated in a transcription of excerpts from the *Grandfather Passage:*

You wished, you wished to know all about my grandfather. Well, he is ne is n-nearly 96, 93 years old. He dresses himself in a old black fox..um.fhrock coat u.. usually s-several buttons missing, yet he sill ooh sill ooh s-sill thinks as whistle..swiftly..as ever.

....his voice is just a bat waxed and squizzers a bit.... he plays sill, sill, skill f-ooh... skillfully and with se.. uh..se..uh..se..sesk u-pon a small organ. Excess, excess, excess, ooh...

In summary, Tim's speech consisted of phoneme additions and deletions and substitution errors which were close approximations of the target sounds. Generally, errors occurred during productions of consonant clusters and multisyllabic words rather than during the production of single phonemes and single syllable words. Visible and audible groping for the correct articulatory postures was apparent. Rate of speech was slow. Apraxia of speech was identified and assigned a severity rating of 4 (7 = most severe rating).

Reading and auditory comprehension were intact. Some spelling errors were present in write-to-dictation tasks. The diagnosis was Broca's Aphasia with coexisting apraxia of speech.

TREATMENT

The Patient's Goals

Treatment sessions were scheduled for 30 minutes daily. At the first session, Tim told me that he was determined to achieve total recovery. He informed me that his goals were the same as before the accident, to return to clinical dentistry in the military, and that he would accept no compromise. With regard to his ability to communicate, Tim stated that he intended to achieve perfect speech.

The Clinician's Goals

Tim was young and highly motivated to excel in treatment. He exhibited mild aphasic and apraxic deficits and was already a functional communicator when he began treatment. His auditory comprehension, reading, and writing were relatively well preserved. His major deficits were in verbal communication, specifically in terms of struggle behavior associated with his apraxia of speech and maintaining a flow of conversation.

The prognosis for improvement was favorable, but it was unclear if this improvement would be sufficient to permit Tim to communicate well enough to practice clinical dentistry. Cousins (1981) has written that, in addition to the primary systems of the human body (e.g., circulatory, digestive, or immune system), the belief system is central to the functioning of the human being. The belief system is a powerful one; it can convert hope and robust expectations into plus factors in rehabilitation and can even go so far as to translate a patient's expectations into physiological change. The clinician is in a position to (a) support the patient's belief system, (b) attempt to alter it, or (c) destroy it. Even though I was not convinced, totally, that Tim would attain his goals, I made the decision to support his belief system, and I accepted his goals.

Controlling Struggle. Treatment involved procedures outlined by Rosenbek (1978) including identifying potential word blocks and errors through (a) recognizing words on which he might have trouble, (b) pausing when his response was not immediately forthcoming or produced correctly, (c) taking time to plan the correct response, and (d) restarting. Tim quickly recognized his difficulties in producing both consonant clusters and words that contained more than one syllable. Soon he was able to anticipate those words on which he blocked or produced errors.

Pausing was more difficult for him. He felt he was "under the gun" to "get the word out" as quickly as he could. A writing-to-dictation task was introduced to facilitate the use of pausing. Multisyllabic words on which he blocked or produced errors in conversation were dictated and he was instructed to write the words leaving spaces between the syllables. Next, he was instructed to read the words aloud, pausing where the spaces occurred. The number of blocks and errors were recorded and Tim was able to track his performance over time. As he watched the number of blocks and errors decrease, he commented that he felt he had "greater control" over his speech and that he found it easier to talk than at any time since the accident.

A secondary benefit was derived from the use of the write-to-dictation task. Tim's spelling improved and he began to correct his spelling errors. This was probably a result of his inspecting each syllable before reading it aloud.

Conversational Practice. Tim's uppermost concern was to be able to communicate well enough to return to his profession. Therefore, treatment was structured so that he could practice strategies to reduce struggle and articulation errors using terms appropriate to clinical dentistry. One issue discussed was the advisability of using x-rays routinely during dental examinations. While arguing that the radiation doses involved were minimal, and therefore not dangerous to the patient, Tim was also practicing anticipating errors, using pauses, planning production, and restarting.

Other topics discussed were dental implants, the benefits of flossing, and dental pathology from a laboratory point of view. Tim and I spoke as two professionals as we discussed issues such as how speech-language pathology relates to dentistry and how we would counsel students who wished to enter our respective fields.

Topics were not restricted to those of a professional nature. We discussed interest rates for buying homes after Tim read aloud from the local newspaper's real estate section. We talked of social events occurring in the city, the rising cost of education, and about skiing. After Tim was allowed weekend passes to spend time in the apartment his wife had rented nearby, we discussed the places they visited while he was on weekend pass.

By the middle of May, the number of errors in Tim's conversational speech had decreased markedly. Results of a readministration of the motor speech evaluation indicated significant improvement in his ability to sequence syllables and a decrease in the incidence of articulatory groping for all tasks. Although apraxia of speech was still identifiable, Tim's overall severity rating was reduced to 2.

Tim was now walking with the aid of a leg brace. His manual dexterity remained too impaired to achieve the precise skills he needed to practice clinical dentistry. Still, he continued to be determined to return to work and was confident that he would do so soon.

A Set-back. In late May an event occurred that lessened Tim's confidence. He suffered a seizure. The seizure was reportedly of the Jacksonian type, a focal seizure that lasted for three minutes. Tim had difficulty moving his right hand for 30 minutes following the episode.

It was obvious that Tim's speech was affected by the seizure. In relating the events before the experience he produced an increasing number of blocks and errors, demonstrating difficulty in sequencing syllables. He began, once again, to practice the programming procedures he had used before.

Redefining Goals. Tim quickly regained the ground he had lost; and for the first time since his accident, he began to consider alternatives to returning to dentistry. In a weekly group session of patients involved in rehabilitation he told the group that he was thinking about possible related lines of work, although he assured them that he was still hoping to return to practicing dentistry once again.

Early in June, Tim announced that he was ready to leave the hospital and "go back to work conducting routine dental exams" at a military base in the city. Although his speech had improved markedly since beginning therapy, he appeared to be unaware of the problems that could confront a dentist with impaired manual dexterity and impaired speech. I asked him several questions: "How will you feel if a child or even an adult says, 'I don't want *him* to be my dentist; his hand looks odd and he talks funny?' Can you handle it if your colleagues do not consult you for your opinions because your speech is not fluent? What will you do? How will you feel?"

Tim lowered his head and looked at the floor. A few moments passed before he answered. Then, in a voice that was barely audible he said, "I-I-I don't know."

Hierarchy of Speaking Situations. To prepare Tim for the transition from communicating in the clinic to communicating in a professional capacity, desensitization techniques (Wolpe, 1958; Brutten & Shoemaker, 1967) were used. Tim was asked to construct a hierarchy of speaking situations in which he could practice talking and to rank-order these situations from least to most fearful. Table 1 shows Tim's hierarchy of increasingly fearful speaking situations.

Next, Tim imagined himself speaking in the situations he had listed, beginning with the least and progressing to the most fearful. As he used

TABLE 2.1
Hierarchy of Fearful Speaking Situations

Speaking with speech clinician

Speaking with members of RMS staff

Speaking with dental hygienist

Lecturing to small group

Lecturing to large group

---

this technique of imaging, he was able to describe the fears he experienced in each situation. Tim reported that "describing the fears made each situation seem less threatening."

Since Tim had become proficient in communicating with his clinician, and this situation was considered least fearful for him, practice in speaking in the hierarchical situations began on step 2, talking informally to the staff on the rehabilitation unit. Tim reported this experience as follows: "It was not too difficult, probably because these people know the 'ins and outs' of my problems."

The next step was speaking to a dental hygienist (whom Tim did not know) in the hospital's dental clinic. In this situation he would need to use terms associated with his profession—many of which were multisyllabic words. Tim reported that the talk went "very well" and that in the 30 minute session he was able to speak with relatively few errors and blocks, especially after the first five minutes. He described his listener as "easy to talk to" and said that when he talked to her, he felt as if he didn't "have to rush to get the words out."

The next situation on the list was one in which Tim was required to give a lecture to a small group. This would be his first opportunity since the accident to speak in a formal situation. He confided that he wanted to teach dentistry some day and that he believed this would be a good chance to try out his ability to lecture.

A series of two formal lectures was arranged with an audience made up of a group of six hospital professionals. Speech-language pathologists, psychologists, and nurses attended the lectures to hear Tim speak on his chosen topic, basic dentistry. There was an interval of several days between the lectures.

Tim's reaction to the first lecture follows:

> I started to speak on what I knew best—dentistry. It was really traumatic. I stumbled over words; I missed words. Coming out of it, I was really upset with myself. I was really frustrated.

Tim practiced imaging between lectures, imagining how he would handle questions and program difficult words. His reaction to his subsequent session was more positive. He said:

> In the second lecture, I did better, and I felt better. I was able to compare my lectures and realize the progress I had made.

Shortly after the lectures Tim received the news that the medical board determining his degree of disability was attempting to declare him 100% disabled. His reaction was intense. "After fighting so hard to regain my speech and the use of my arm and leg, it looks as if I won't be able to return to the military after all." He vowed to appeal the decision, if it was made. "It's so unfair," he said, "the people who I worked so hard for just want to pitch me out. After five years, they just want to wash their hands of me."

Tim was discharged from the hospital near the end of June. He went to work in the dental clinic on a nearby military base. In November, he and his wife consented to come to the local university so that Tim could talk to a group of students and practicing speech-language pathologists. Thus, he was ready to attempt the last step in the hierarchy—that of "speaking to a large group."

The following excerpts are taken from Tim's talk at the meeting. His comments reflect an aphasic patient's feelings about what it is like to be aphasic.

ON THE INABILITY TO UNDERSTAND SPEECH:

> I went through a time where I was hearing things that people did *not* say. I would swear that Nan said something which she claimed she had not said. I still do this, sometimes.

ON HOW IT FEELS TO BE UNABLE TO TALK:

> Something that really irritated me was that soon after surgery, there were some not too bright people who were talking down to *me*! They couldn't imagine that my mind was still good; they thought my whole rational process and my ability to think were all gone, because I couldn't talk.

ON LISTENER "FILL-IN"

> There were times when I would begin a sentence and, then, couldn't think of the word I needed to finish it. I understand that some people were not familiar with my speech problems and were trying to help by finishing my thoughts. Some of my close relatives did this. I wish they would have given me more time to express my thoughts.

ON PREPARING THE PATIENT FOR THE REACTION OF HIS LISTENERS:

It is important in your job to prepare a patient for the reaction other people may have to his speech, and to desensitize him to that reaction. In my case, I wanted to be a practicing dentist, again. When I left the hospital, I was put into a situation where I was no longer being sheltered. People usually don't feel too good about going to the dentist, anyway, but when they see a dentist who can't talk, or sounds funny when he does talk, they really react in a negative way. So desensitization was really important for me.

ON PERSONAL GOALS:

At first, I wanted total recovery. I wanted to be the same as I was before the accident. It took me a while to realize that I would have limitations. Now I know what my limitations are.

ON THE IMPORTANCE OF THE APHASIA CLINICIAN IN THE REHABILITATION PROCESS:

There is so much you can do in addition to teaching the patient to talk. The patient's emotional side should be considered equally as important as his speech. I always saw my clinician as someone I could communicate with who would wait for me to talk. This is so important—to wait for the person to "get out" whatever he needs to say ...

We were ... not just one professional instructing and one patient learning, but two professionals working together. It really made a big difference, not just in my speech, but in me, because I felt not like "just a patient" but a person with dignity.

You can make a total difference in a patient's life. Don't take your job lightly. I just feel ... Dr. Vogel basically saved my life, because if I couldn't talk, couldn't speak well, I could have developed all sorts of emotional problems. Really, take what you do very, very seriously because you can make such a difference for your patients.

In this final and most feared speaking situation, Tim was assigned a rating of *1* (minimal impairment, in terms of his apraxia of speech, and most listeners would have judged his speech to be normal.

Follow-up. Several months after the university presentation, Tim returned to the clinic. He reported that he had been given official permission to return to permanent active military duty. After two appeals, the medical board was convinced that he could remain in the military practicing his profession. Tim was still using the leg brace and his manual dexterity remained mildly impaired. He was concerned that although the staff at the dental clinic had tried to be understanding and helpful, he had been allowed to participate only in routine examinations. He felt his talents weren't being utilized fully. "Still," he affirmed, "I achieved my goal. I'm a practicing dentist again."

One year later, Tim visited the clinic again. This time he reported that he had been reassigned to duty in the southeastern United States. "There is a university near the base," he said. "I plan to take some courses in computer programming. Who knows? Maybe I'll begin a new career." Before he left, we spoke of his move and his plans, focusing on the future. "I came here to thank you," he told me. "Thank you for helping me to help myself."

Postscript

Tim's case illustrates the wisdom of Schuell, Jenkins, and Jiminez-Pabon (1964) who suggested that when the aphasic patient believes he is ready to return to work, the clinician should be more inclined to accept the patient's judgment rather than the results of standardized tests. Perhaps more importantly, it shows a need to make room in the caseload for the minimally impaired aphasic patient, who with assistance, might achieve goals such as Tim's.

REFERENCES

Brutten, E., & Shoemaker, D. (1967). *The modification of stuttering.* Englewood Cliffs, NJ: Prentice Hall.

Cousins, N. (1981). *Human options. An autobiographic notebook.* New York: W.W. Norton.

Goodglass. H., & Kaplan, E. (1972). *The assessment of aphasia and related disorders.* Philadelphia: Lea & Febiger.

Rosenbek, J.C. (1978). Treating apraxia of speech. In D.F. Johns (Ed.), *Clinical management of neurogenic communication disorders.* Boston: Little, Brown.

Rosenbek, J.C., Lemme, M.L., Ahern, M.B., Harris, E.H., & Wertz, R.T. (1973). A treatment for apraxia of speech in adults. *Journal of Speech and Hearing Disorders, 38,* 462–472.

Schuell. H., & Jenkins. J.J., & Jimenez-Pabon, E. (1964). *Aphasia in adults: Diagnosis, prognosis, and treatment.* New York: Harper and Row.

Sklar, M. (1966). *Sklar Aphasia Scale.* Beverly Hills, CA: Western Psychological Services.

Wepman, J. (1978). Aphasia therapy: A new look. *Journal of Speech and Hearing Disorders, 37,* 203–213.

Wolpe, J. (1978). *Psychotherapy by reciprocol inhibition.* Stanford, CA: Stanford University Press.

CHAPTER 3
Beyond Our Usual Treatment Goals: Treatment of a High Level Aphasic Person
Marie T. Rau

> Rau demonstrates the value of providing speech and language treatment and counseling to high level aphasic clients even after they have regained "functional communication." She describes a program designed to ameliorate specific deficits and to prepare a client for return to work as a college teacher. Follow-up and continuous evaluation of speech and language performance in social and vocational settings by client and clinician alike constituted important aspects of treatment.
>
> 1. How does Rau involve the client's wife in the treatment program? What is the value of this procedure? To the wife? To the client?
> 2. What are some of the sensitive counseling issues regarding the client's feelings about himself and his communication that arise during the course of treatment? How are these issues dealt with by the author?
> 3. What limitations do standardized tests have in evaluating the results of treatment in cases similar to the one presented by Rau? How does the author conduct treatment sessions designed to prepare the client to return to college teaching? How does Rau evaluate the results of this treatment?
> 4. Does the long-term follow-up provided this high level client have therapeutic value? Why or why not?

BACKGROUND INFORMATION

Dr. Robert Wilson, 52, was a right-handed man who had suffered a left-hemisphere cerebrovascular accident of sudden onset in June 1982, with resulting aphasia. His native language was English, and at the time of the stroke he was employed full-time as a chemistry professor in a small college. His entire adult career had been spent in academic settings, in teaching, research, and administration. Dr. Wilson was married and had two adult children, the youngest of whom, a son, had recently moved back home.

Medical History

On June 2, 1982, Dr. Wilson went to the medical out-patient clinic of a private hospital complaining of weakness and dyspnea which had been present for about a month. He had a known history of cardiac disease. An echocardiogram in 1981 had shown mitral valve prolapse, and since 1980 he had experienced paroxysmal atrial flutter. The client had undergone coronary artery bypass surgery in December 1981 related to persistent angina. During that year he also had suffered transient ischemic attacks (TIAs) involving blurred vision, right arm weakness, and vertigo conditions which cleared after a few hours.

After examination in the clinic on June 2, an echocardiogram was scheduled and performed later that day at another private hospital. While undergoing the echocardiogram, Dr. Wilson abruptly became aphasic, with right-sided facial weakness and right arm weakness noted. A computerized tomography (CT) scan performed shortly after this episode was normal. He was then transferred back to the private hospital operated by his health insurance plan, where he was observed to be able to "say a few words." His right arm strength had improved, but mild right facial and arm weakness were still noted. Over the course of a two week hospital stay, the right arm and facial weakness resolved spontaneously and completely. His aphasia improved gradually and progressively, but Dr. Wilson was described as still having a "moderate aphasic deficit" at the time of hospital discharge. The final neurological diagnosis was a stroke involving a probable embolism to the distribution of the left middle cerebral artery. The etiology of the presumed embolism remained unknown at discharge. The echocardiogram showed no evidence of an intracardiac clot. A digital cerebral angiogram performed on June 16, 1982 showed "wide open" carotid arteries, with no evidence of stenosis and no other clinically obvious intracerebral arterial disease. Dr. Wilson's early postoperative recovery from the stroke and initial rehabilitation efforts were interrupted when he experienced a myocardial infarction two days after the stroke. His recovery from the heart attack was uneventful, and Dr. Wilson was discharged home 15 days after the occurrence of the stroke.

SPEECH AND LANGUAGE EVALUATION

Acute Care Hospital

The initial speech and language evaluation was completed by the speech-language pathologist who saw Dr. Wilson in the acute-care hospital. Her report indicated a "moderate fluent aphasia crossing all receptive and expressive language modalities." In an initial administration of the *Token Test* (DeRenzi & Vignolo, 1962), the client made 27 errors on a 45 item version of the test. At first, Dr. Wilson was seen three times weekly while in the hospital, with "significant improvements in speech-language functioning noted." His communicative status at discharge from the private hospital was described in the progress notes with the comment: Residual fluent aphasia persists. On the *Token Test*, an improvement in performance from 27 errors to only 15 errors was noted. With regard to other aspects of auditory comprehension, the client made no errors on simple, one-step commands; he showed the most difficulty on two-step, "semi-complex" instructions. There was evidence of noise build-up (Brookshire, 1976) on auditory processing tasks. Dr. Wilson was observed to make occasional use of "reauditorization" (Schuell, 1953) to facilitate comprehension. Reading skills showed a similar pattern to auditory comprehension performance, with breakdowns occurring with increased length and complexity of the written material. Expressive language was characterized by: (a) beginning evidence of self monitoring of verbal errors, with frequent successful efforts at correcting them; (b) fluent verbalizations, often containing superfluous utterances that decreased the preciseness with which the client communicated his thoughts; (c) word substitutions, sometimes semantically related; and (d) decreased use of nouns and verbs. Written language expression was characterized by legible attempts at target words, but with errors similar to those seen in verbal output noted, as well as frequent, phonetically related spelling errors. Given the rapid amount of improvement related to spontaneous recovery that the client had already made, it was felt by the clinician that Dr. Wilson showed good prognosis for further improvement in communication skills, and it was recommended that he continue to be seen in language treatment two to three times a week. Because his health insurance coverage did not include outpatient speech and language treatment, Dr. Wilson was referred by his clinician to the Portland VA Medical Center to continue his communication rehabilitation.

Portland Veterans Administration Medical Center

The client was first seen at this facility on June 21, 1982. The *Porch Index of Communicative Ability* (Porch, 1967) was administered on July 1, 1982, at one month postonset, with the following results: Dr. Wilson achieved an overall score of 13.59, which placed him at the 84th percentile in a large, random sample of left hemisphere damaged adults. Examination of PICA test results indicated that he had most problems with the two most difficult subtests on the battery: formulating complete sentences verbally about the functions of test objects (subtest I) and formulating complete written sentences about the functions of test items (subtest A). While overall PICA performance indicated his aphasic deficits to be in the mild range, decreased efficiency of communication across all language modalities was noted. This reduced efficiency of communication was reflected in processing delays, requests for repetition of the stimulus, self-corrections, and some incomplete responses. Few frank errors were noted except for spelling errors on the graphic subtests.

In conversational interactions during the evaluation phase, Dr. Wilson would occasionally show that he was having difficulty processing auditory information; at such times, his responses reflected misunderstanding or incomplete understanding of the clinician's comment or question. Expressive language was characterized by frequent word-finding difficulties, semantic errors, and reduction in the use of specific content words. In conversational discourse, his frequent failure to use referents (persons' names, names of places or things) made it difficult to follow the thread of conversation.

Another aspect of Dr. Wilson's communicative behavior was the extreme embarrassment he showed when even a slight communicative breakdown occurred. He would frequently apologize and berate himself for pauses and word-retrieval problems, and interpret any question asked by the clinician—even one asked purely for further information or conversational stimulation—as reflecting some "mistake" he had made. In summary, this warm, pleasant, and intelligent man who had already regained a relatively high level of functional communication at one month postonset, was exhibiting a greatly reduced self-image and a considerable lack of self-confidence related to his verbal performance.

STAGES OF TREATMENT

Ameliorating Specific Deficits

Goals. Early treatment goals directly related to assisting Dr. Wilson in improving his communicative efficiency centered around word-retrieval problems, his inefficient and somewhat "rambling" verbal and written communication, and spelling errors. Because of the mild nature of his aphasia and a strong desire to contribute to his own rehabilitation program and to manage his own recovery, his input was utilized in determining both treatment goals and specific activities. He expressed the desire to have his wife participate by sitting in on early sessions; this gave the clinician an opportunity to model optimum ways of communicating with Dr. Wilson and of reacting to his communicative breakdowns, as well as for dealing with counseling issues as they came up during the course of treatment. Dr. Wilson also expressed the desire to have treatment sessions focus on conversational practice, with structured word-retrieval activities, both verbal and written, saved for home practice.

Structure. Treatment sessions were scheduled for one to one and a half hours twice weekly. Mrs. Wilson drove her husband to the clinic for these early meetings and sat in on almost all treatment sessions for the first few months. While this might have been detrimental to some clients, such an intensive level of spouse participation proved extremely beneficial in this situation. Mrs. Wilson, a highly intelligent, sensitive, and supportive person, contributed in a positive way to her husband's rehabilitation. This was probably in no small part due to her background in counseling, as well as to the couple's close personal relationship. Dr. Wilson appeared to enjoy having his wife present, and did not unduly depend on her to communicate for him. In fact, he would occasionally remind the clinician and his spouse that it was he who was there to do most of the talking!

Procedures and Materials. Because Dr. Wilson had expressed a strong preference for conversational practice during clinic treatment time, and because the mild nature of his aphasic deficits warranted such a conversational emphasis, two basic approaches described in the literature on aphasia treatment were employed. One such approach Wepman (1972) called "indirect therapy" or "thought-centered" therapy. This approach involves focusing on appropriate speaker-listener roles to convey intended messages or meanings, rather than on linguistic accuracy per se. Wepman's approach concentrates on the thoughts and ideas underlying verbal messages, and depends upon speaker-listener exchanges to formulate, perceive, and revise intended messages until consensus about their meaning is reached (Martin, 1981). During the treatment session, this is accomplished by the clinician reflecting back to the client his or her intended thoughts, by paraphrasing the client's intended message, and by keeping the conversation "on track" when word retrieval problems have resulted in communication breakdown.

A second approach which seemed appropriate to employ in treatment of Dr. Wilson has been described by Davis and Wilcox (1981). This approach is known as "Promoting Aphasics' Communicative Effectiveness," or PACE. This treatment approach also emphasizes the roles of speaker and listener, the pragmatic context of the communication, and the exchange or transfer of information rather than linguistic or phonemic accuracy. PACE thus incorporates elements of natural conversation into aphasia treatment (Davis & Wilcox, 1981). In particular, the interaction between clinician and client in PACE is based on "the main objective of participants in conversation, that being to convey messages consisting of new information" (Davis & Wilcox, 1981, p. 172).

As can be seen from the above descriptions of the treatment approaches adopted for this client, there is considerable overlap between Wepman's indirect, or communication-centered approach, and PACE. Elements of both theoretical approaches were incorporated into Dr. Wilson's program. For example, all of the information communicated by Dr. Wilson when he assumed the speaker role was "new information" to the clinician, in the sense that stimuli were either thoughts and ideas the client wanted to express, or materials such as articles or pictures related to his work that Dr. Wilson himself brought in (rather than clinician-selected pictures or printed verbal stimuli). Conversational topics included hobbies and interests (music, travel, home remodeling projects in which the client was engaged), work-related topics such as personal research, a book he had planned to write, college gossip, and current events. Treatment procedures employed within this conversational context included providing target words (when known) if Dr. Wilson indicated he needed assistance, asking questions for clarification, and rephrasing or paraphrasing information exchanged in an effort to keep the conversation on track.

Independent activities during this initial stage of treatment included reading, writing, and vocabulary retrieval activities. Two very useful sources of home practice material were the *Workbook for Aphasia* (Brubaker, 1978) and the *Mammoth Book of Word Games* (Manchester, 1976). Activities included selecting synonyms, antonyms, and associated words; coming up with synonyms, antonyms, and associated words; listing multiple meanings of words; writing sentences using target words; unscrambling syllables and words; following written directions; and solving word puzzles. Goals for these activities included not only increasing accuracy of spelling and word selection, and improving the clarity and conciseness of written sentences, but also decreasing the time it took to complete these workbook exercises. Initially, it would take Dr. Wilson forty-five minutes or an hour to complete a workbook page. He found it reinforcing to keep track of the beginning and ending time of an activity, and to see that he was improving in both speed and accuracy.

Toward the end of the first six months of treatment Dr. Wilson suggested that he wanted to work on regaining his reading facility. Some initial attempts on his own to read scientific journals had proved devastating when he discovered he could no longer grasp once familiar details, even with several readings. Short articles from lay publications on science, such as *Discovery* and *Science 82,* proved to be more appropriate for renewing reading skills. As he progressed and regained confidence, Dr. Wilson would bring in articles from *Science* and the *New England Journal of Medicine* which he and the clinician would read independently and then discuss.

Counseling. An integral part of every treatment session with the Wilsons during the early phases of therapy was counseling. Questions and concerns at first focused on information about strokes, and physiological and behavioral changes related to a stroke. Dr. Wilson was particularly distressed about his apparent lack of control over his emotions and the frequent crying spells he experienced. To him this was a source of great embarrassment and concern. He would verbalize his reluctance to attend public and social functions because of his emotional lability. This occurred at a time when his recovering language skills would have benefited from more social interaction. Counseling Dr. Wilson about the nature of what Lieberman and Benson (1977) have termed "hyperactive emotional reflexes" following a stroke, and discussing possible ways of dealing with moments of lability only partially alleviated his concerns. On more than one occasion, he stated that uncontrolled crying or feeling that he was about to cry was the most distressing aspect of the stroke. With time, even up to a year and a half after the stroke, both the evidence of emotional lability and Dr. Wilson's reaction to his reduced emotional control diminished.

Both of the Wilsons read and gained encouragement from a book by Arthur Freese (1980), *Stroke: The New Hope and the New Help.* Selected personal accounts of recovery after a stroke with aphasia (Buck, 1968; Moss, 1972; Wulf, 1973) were also useful in providing information and insight to the Wilsons. This bibliotherapy also served as the basis for several discussions during counseling sessions as the Wilsons would ask questions or share their reaction to something they had read.

Other concerns that became the focus of counseling involved Dr. Wilson's perceptions of how others now viewed him as a speaker. He expressed his feelings and observations that family members and friends now "talked down" to him, as if he couldn't understand, and that they provided frequent repetitions, even when he didn't ask for them. He was particularly distressed that his adult son, who had a degree in psychology, seemed to have lost respect for him because of his communication difficulties. Although Dr. Wilson at this time still was making only infrequent contacts with colleagues at the college, he sensed that these fellow professionals felt "uncomfortable" around him and that they quickly terminated any conversational exchanges when he attended a social event or dropped by to pick up his mail. Dealing with these issues as they came up during treatment involved discussing why some people might be responding in these ways. We also encouraged Dr. Wilson to share with his close friends and family members how he felt about them repeating themselves unnecessarily and simplifying their explanations and vocabulary. At the same time, he was encouraged to ask for clarification and further explanation when he felt that he had missed some aspect of a conversational exchange. It proved very helpful to have Dr. Wilson's wife participate in these counseling sessions, as she became sensitized to his feelings about his changed status as a communicator.

Perhaps most important of all, early counseling regarding the aims of treatment and the progress observed provided the Wilsons with, in their words, "hope and encouragement" that return to meaningful work was a reasonable goal. They related later in treatment how devastated they were when a neurologist gave them a very early negative prognosis and suggested to Mrs. Wllson that she place her husband in a nursing home.

Results. Objective testing showed gradual improvement in communicative efficiency. A PICA administered at three months postonset (September 1982) indicated improvement in the Overall score from the 84th to the 90th percentile. Largest gains were on subtest I and graphic test A, the formulating of verbal and written sentences about the test objects. Dr. Wilson's improved efficiency in dealing with auditory information was reflected in improved performance on subtests IX, VI, X, and D, all heavily dependent on auditory processing. Evidence of a possible "noise build-up" effect was still seen, however, in that Dr. Wilson achieved a higher score on spontaneously writing the names of objects (Graphic test B) than he did when the names were presented (Graphic test C), or when the names were spelled for him (Graphic test D). Subsequent follow-up PICA tests remained at or about the 90th percentile, indicating both a ceiling effect of the PICA in ability to measure further gains made by Dr. Wilson, and some remaining inefficiencies in terms of delays, self-corrections, and occasional grammatic and spelling errors in written communication.

A *Token Test* administered at six months postonset revealed only five errors on a 62 item version of the test, a performance almost within the range of normal (Wertz, Keith, & Custer, 1971). As was the case with the PICA, subsequent administrations of the *Token Test* showed stability of performance on this measure at about five errors.

Subjectively, at the end of six months of treatment, Dr. Wilson had improved significantly in the facility and specificity with which he could retrieve and use words. He showed both increasing awareness of his off-target word selection and a greater tolerance for his occasional word retrieval problems. He reported that reading was going easily and that he felt that he was ready to resume some involvement in professional activities. Both the progress that the client had made and his desire to begin preparing to get back to his teaching and research led us into the next phase of treatment.

Preparation for Return to Work

Goals. In the early spring of 1983, Dr. Wilson announced at the beginning of a treatment session that he had informed the college he would be able to return to part-time teaching in the fall. He was scheduled to teach one course. It was a basic course in his particular area of expertise and one that he had taught several times previously. Thus, throughout that summer and early fall, treatment sessions focused on the goal of preparing Dr. Wilson for resuming teaching and related academic responsibilities. The client brought another goal to this phase of treatment as well. He began gathering material for a book he had been planning to write for many years. It was to be a book written for lay audiences about the contributions and applications of chemistry to the advancement of knowledge in many areas of science. Preparation of an outline for this book became a second language treatment goal during this period.

Procedures. During the summer and early fall of 1983, treatment sessions focused on the actual textbook material Dr. Wilson would be covering in his class, using the book that he had chosen for the course. To prepare for an instructional session, I would read a chapter or portion of a chapter and Dr. Wilson would prepare a lecture about the topic to be discussed. I assumed the role of a student during these sessions, asking questions for clarification and indicating when a particular idea was not clearly presented. This preparation phase served the purpose of assisting Dr. Wilson to organize course materials and to prepare outlines of the material to be covered in class lectures. It also provided him with practice in expressing complex concepts in a less demanding setting than the actual classroom. The hospital library proved to be a valuable resource in providing slides and other audiovisual teaching aids that Dr. Wilson was able to use in his preparatory lectures. Although he had previously taught the course for which we were rehearsing, the acquisition of new supplementary teaching aids such as the slides appeared to give Dr. Wilson confidence and to help him to organize his lectures. They also allowed him to compensate for some of the inefficiencies in his verbal expression.

Other activities were also beneficial during these months before he went back to teaching. Although most activities were arranged or suggested by Dr. Wilson himself, I encouraged and reinforced these out-of-the-clinic activities. For example, Dr. Wilson expressed an interest in visiting some of the basic science research labs within the medical center, and tours of the various research facilities were arranged. At the same time, he began volunteering a few hours a week of his time at a nearby regional research facility where he knew a number of the faculty. He also resumed attending department seminars and faculty meetings at the college. All of these activities appeared to increase his confidence and to improve his self image. Dr. Wilson was particularly pleased to be asked to serve as the outside member on two master's thesis committees during this phase of treatment, and to successfully complete these responsibilities.

Meanwhile, through these six months of treatment, Dr. Wilson made some progress on his book. He made verbal and written contact with several people across the country, and also made many trips to obtain information for his book. These contacts were often difficult, as he would worry about whether he was making himself clear, or whether he was explaining his plan for the book in a coherent way. Still, he persisted.

Counseling. As Dr. Wilson prepared to resume his teaching responsibilities and step back into his professional life, counseling became more directly focused on compensatory strategies such as modification of work schedules and time tables for accomplishing tasks. He also began to frequently express concern regarding how much he should tell colleagues and students about his stroke and communication difficulties. He was also having problems dealing with limitations related to fatigue and reduced language efficiency. As he pursued the many activities outlined above, there was a sense that he was constantly testing himself to determine whether he could still perform at his former intellectual level. Balancing and defining my counseling role in working with this high-level client was challenging and difficult during this phase of treatment. For example, if I had suggested that Dr. Wilson reduce the demands of his daily schedule before he experienced frustration and, at times, outright failure, my advice would have been promptly rejected. These and other sensitive issues, such as allowing himself more time for rest, could only be discussed and possible solutions suggested when the client himself brought the problems up.

Follow-up

Goals. In the fall of 1983, Dr. Wilson returned to the classroom on a part-time basis. He had expressed a strong desire to continue our twice-weekly meetings until he saw how the teaching was going to go, and it seemed important to do so. Treatment goals during this follow-up phase were directly related to evaluating whether teaching was a realistic and reasonable endeavor for Dr. Wilson to pursue, and what further assistance he might need if he was to again teach successfully.

Procedures. With the return to classroom lecturing, one procedure that worked quite successfully was to have Dr. Wilson tape record lectures and bring the tapes to our treatment sessions. There, he and I would listen to and critique the presentations for clarity, for logical thought flow, and for the success with which Dr. Wilson handled students' questions. We continued to use our meetings to have him practice lecture material and to deal with specific problems in the work setting as they arose.

One problem was spelling. It embarrassed Dr. Wilson when he would misspell technical and scientific terms as he attempted to put them on the board, or when he would be unable to recall the spelling of certain words under the pressure of the moment. After a few of these negative experiences, he adopted the suggested strategy of preparing overhead transparencies at his leisure so he could check or look up the spelling of difficult words beforehand. It also facilitated the flow of his lectures to have outlines of the main points to be covered on transparencies or handouts. He gradually began to appreciate that he now needed these teaching aids, whereas prior to the stroke it had not been "his style."

Another problem was the formulating of quiz questions and examinations. After some student bewilderment over a few of his examination questions, Dr. Wilson began to prepare his tests early and bring them to therapy where we could critique them together.

A very useful source of feedback information was the end-of-quarter student evaluation form. Student comments in general gave Dr. Wilson "satisfactory" to "good" ratings in various aspects of teaching, although it appeared they interpreted his occasional word-finding problems and reduced verbal efficiency as lack of preparation and organization. We were able to use these student evaluations to help set goals for the next quarter's teaching.

Counseling. Several counseling issues underscored the importance of keeping a follow-up contact with this high-level client after he returned to work. For example, we discussed at length whether he should attempt to return to full-time teaching or continue with a part-time work load. It was my strong feeling that a full-time teaching load would be too much for Dr. Wilson, because of the greatly increased amount of time it took him to prepare lectures, examinations, and correspondence.

Another counseling issue involved the scheduling and content of some of his assigned classes. During the spring term, he was assigned a class to teach in the early evenings, in a subject area with which he was only somewhat familiar. This proved to be very difficult and frustrating because of fatigue at that hour of the day and the complexity of the subject matter.

Results. The results were mixed in terms of how successful Dr. Wilson had been in the first year of his return to classroom teaching. He had experienced some success in teaching two courses in his particular area of expertise when he adopted compensatory strategies and teaching aids. On the other hand, he had felt frustration and failure in his attempt to teach less familiar material under less than optimum conditions. He also had to deal with pressure from the college and his department to consider early retirement.

At this time, Dr. Wilson is on a year's medical leave. He continues to work on improving his language abilities with the goal of returning to part-time teaching next fall. He continues to improve in his writing facility through practice on a personal home computer. He is also able to read technical articles with more efficiency. He is becoming much more realistic in his assessment of what he can and cannot do and how he might utilize compensatory strategies to overcome his remaining language deficits.

CONCLUSIONS: WHAT CAN BE LEARNED FROM THIS CASE?

Dr. Wilson's treatment history offers several important lessons. First, the mild nature of his aphasia and his prolonged treatment program challenged the clinician to grapple with some of the important issues raised by Wertz (1978) in his summary of a round table discussion on the treatment of mild aphasia: For how long should treatment be continued after the client is a "functional" communicator? For how long should treatment be continued after PICA scores have plateaued? In this case, becoming a functional communicator in the world at large and reaching the 90th percentile on the PICA did *not* mean reaching a truly functional level in the verbally demanding job of college teaching, nor did reaching these goals mean that Dr. Wilson would make no further gains in language facility. It was important and justifiable that his rehabilitation continue beyond these "usual treatment goals."

A second valuable insight provided by this case is the recognition that clients and their families may initially come to therapy with an inappropriate initial prognosis, a prognosis that may be negative and inordinately pessimistic. Realistic goal setting and early demonstration of progress in such cases can serve to alleviate the all too common misconception that treatment "won't help."

Another important lesson to be learned from this case is the critical importance of providing support and follow-up in the form of clinician contact during that transition period from the clinic back to the real world of a verbal occupation. Even if the frequency of treatment is reduced, regularly scheduled follow-up sessions can be utilized to work through difficulties and obtain feedback about what is working for the client, and what still needs shoring up.

A third lesson from this case involves the *timing* of the acceptance of communicative limitations following a stroke. For some persons, an early verdict of "You really won't be able to return to your former work" will be neither accepted nor adhered to. Dr. Wilson needed to go back to teaching in order to experience his stroke-related limitations, and to come to accept the need for some compensatory strategies and adjustment in work load, scheduling, and time allowed for completing certain tasks. Until he had returned to the classroom and experienced some frustrations himself, my suggestions about reducing his schedule, preparing detailed lecture notes ahead of time, and allowing several days to prepare written examinations were politely listened to, but just as politely rejected. There is an individually determined time when each person who has experienced the losses that a stroke represents is ready to accept the necessary adjustments and adaptations that will allow them to continue on with their lives. It does not appear that this process can be significantly shortened by counseling.

REFERENCES

Brookshire. R.H. (1976). Differences in responding to auditory verbal materials among aphasic patients. *Acta Symbolica, 5,* 1–18.

Brubaker, S.H. (1978). *Workbook for Aphasia*. Detroit: Wayne State University Press.

Buck, M. (1968). *Dysphasia: Professional guidance for family and patient.* Englewood Cliffs. NJ: Prentice-Hall.

Davis, G.A., & Wilcox. M.J. (1981). Incorporating parameters of natural conversation in aphasia treatment. In R. Chapey (Ed.), *Language intervention strategies in adult aphasia*. Baltimore: Williams & Wilkins.

DeRenzi, E., & Vignolo, L.A. (1962). The Token Test: A sensitive test to detect receptive disturbances in aphasia. *Brain, 85,* 665–678.

Freese, A. (1980). *Stroke: The new hope and new help*. New York: Random House.

Lieberman, A., & Benson, D.F. (1977). Control of emotional expression in pseudobulbar palsy. *Archives of Neurology, 34,* 717–719.

Manchester. R.B. (1976). *The mammoth book of word games*. New York: Hart Publishing.

Martin, A.D. (1981). An examination of Wepman's thought centered therapy. In: R. Chapey (Ed.). *Language intervention strategies in adult aphasia*. Baltimore: Williams & Wilkins.

Moss, C.S. (1972). *Recovery with aphasia: The aftermath of my stroke*. Urbana, IL: University of Illinois Press.

Porch, B.E. (1967). *Porch Index of Communicative Ability*. Palo Alto, CA: Consulting Psychologists Press.

Schuell, H. (1953). Auditory impairment in aphasia: Significance and retraining techniques. *Journal of Speech and Hearing Disorders, 18,* 14–21.

Wepman, J., 1972). Aphasia therapy: A new look. *Journal of Speech and Hearing Disorders, 37,* 203–214.

Wertz, R.T. (1978). Treating mildly aphasic patients: A round table discussion. In R. Brookshire (Ed.), *Clinical Aphasiology Conference Proceedings.* Minneapolis: BRK Publishers.

Wertz, R.T., Keith, R.L., & Custer, D.D. (1971, November). Normal and aphasic behavior on a measure of auditory input and a measure of verbal output. Paper presented at the Annual Convention of the American Speech-Language and Hearing Association, Chicago, IL.

Wulf, H.H. (1978). *Aphasia, my world alone.* Detroit: Wayne State University Press.

CHAPTER 4
A Spouse's Role in Rehabilitation
Elizabeth J. Webster

> Webster's contribution underscores the fact that aphasia is a family problem and that the patient's significant others warrant assistance and guidance in coping with the disorder. She describes the recovery of functional communication by a severely aphasic man through changes in the feelings, attitudes and perceptions of the client's wife over a two-year treatment course. The author clearly illustrates the importance of counseling, socialization and group support in aphasia rehabilitation.
>
> 1. What behaviors of the client's wife (Cora) might have been counterproductive to rehabilitation efforts? How did the client (Lou) react to these behaviors? What may have prompted Cora to respond to her husband's deficits in this fashion? What was the nature of the couple's relationship before the stroke? Immediately after the stroke? At the end of therapy?
> 2. What does Webster mean when she refers to Cora's ambivalence and her inability to let go?
> 3. In the course of Lou's treatment, Cora eventually accepted (a) the fact that Lou would drive again and (b) that he would need to use an augmentative device to communicate. How did this acceptance influence Lou's speech and language recovery? What were the benefits Cora received?
> 4. In two years of treatment Lou improved his PICA scores negligibly. What are some of the improvements he made that could not be measured by the PICA? How might these influence his life? Cora's life? Was the therapeutic effort to prompt these changes justified? Why or why not?
> 5. For information relative to the counseling of aphasic families the reader is referred to the works of Newhoff and Davis (1978), Linebaugh and Young-Charles (1978), Chwat and Gurland (1981), Webster and Newhoff (1981), Webster, Dans, and Sanders (1982), and Davis (1983) at the end of this chapter.

Introduction

If the sole measure of successful treatment of aphasia is the client's improvement in use of speech, this is a story of failure. If, however, improved functional communication and a closer relationship between client and spouse are among criteria for success, then counseling with Cora and treatment for her aphasic husband, Lou, were successful. This couple was seen for two years in a university clinic as they struggled to repair their damaged lives and to create from the pieces a new but productive relationship.

The primary focus here is on Cora. She was a regular and very verbal participant in group counseling sessions conducted for spouses at the time their aphasic partners were enrolled for speech-language therapy. A speech-language pathologist with training and experience in counseling met with the spouse group for one hour a week throughout each semester the aphasic clients were seen. Because these groups were used for student training as well to provide a service, each semester one or two advanced graduate students participated in all sessions. Thus the group's composition varied slightly each semester, making possible new as well as continuing supportive friendships between participants. The story of Cora and Lou is told primarily through Cora's discussion. Her contributions are supplemented by clinicians' observations of Cora in the group, Cora's reports of her interactions with Lou, and by clinical reports of Lou's therapy.

THE CASE: CORA AND LOU

Early Observations of Cora

Cora was a short, remarkably obese, round-faced, good-natured looking woman who appeared to smile almost constantly. She laughingly introduced herself as "living proof of the old saying, 'laugh and grow fat.'" The spouse group met in a room furnished with a sofa and arm chairs. On the occasion of the first group meeting Cora glanced at the furnishings and said, "There's nowhere I can sit where I wouldn't get stuck or where I'd be able to get up." The clinicians quickly learned to provide Cora with a straight chair that would accommodate her bulk.

Despite her smile, Cora often appeared pale, short of breath, and moved slowly and wearily. She spoke of a continuing problem with angina that limited her activity. She also reported that she was under medical treatment for coronary disease.

Cora quickly established herself as an asset to the spouse program. Whereas most of the spouses directed their early statements and questions to the group leader, Cora distributed hers among all participants.

Although Cora laughed often as she related her current problems and feelings, she seemed to speak of them openly and honestly. Furthermore, she did not laugh as others detailed their difficulties. She listened to others and responded with understanding as they expressed their emotions.

Cora's Reports of Life with Lou

Family members of aphasic individuals usually begin their group discussions by sharing details of events surrounding the affected individual's acquisition of impairment. Likewise, Cora and the people in her group discussed details of their spouses' strokes as they understood and remembered them. Cora reported that Lou had a "very big" CVA with right hemiplegia and both receptive and expressive aphasia. Now, a year after Lou's stroke, Cora judged him to be completely helpless. She insisted he use a wheelchair and refused to let him try to walk, even when aided by his heavy leg brace and walker. She fed him his meals and interpreted his polysyllabic jargon. Lou's "crying jags" distressed her and she was bewildered and often angered by his displays of anger and frustration. Cora attributed Lou's crying and anger to the post-stroke personality changes she had read about. When clinicians had suggested that Lou needed to be more independent, Cora had quickly countered with numerous reasons that his greater independence would make her life harder. For example, she did not know what she would do if Lou fell while trying to walk and she felt she couldn't trust him to make "reasonable" judgments.

Typically, as group members discuss their spouses' current problems and their strategies for coping with new and strange relationships, they also reveal much about their previous life situations. Thus Cora spoke of Lou as having been very bright, assertive, "determined and dominating." She said, "He ruled the roost at home and made all the decisions for me and the two children." She said Lou, an engineer, had risen to an important executive position in a large midwestern corporation. "He was like that (dominating) in his job, too, and nobody went against his wishes."

Cora related that Lou had a history of diabetes. He had also suffered two heart attacks, the second of which "scared him enough to convince him to retire from his pressure-cooker job." After he retired Lou decided that he and Cora would move to the South to live with Cora's mother, a semi-invalid. Despite Cora's protests and resentments the couple moved in with the mother. Cora reported that she put off the move as long as possible, saying, "I really dragged my feet till Lou got mad. He gave me a deadline and told me he was moving on that date with me or without me. I got busy and we sold the house. I cried all the time I was packing." But she laughed as she related the story. Cora did not know Lou's motivation for wishing to live with her mother because, "We really didn't discuss anything very much. The more I asked him why he wanted to live with a demanding old lady, the more he refused to talk about it."

Cora hated living with her mother. Part of Cora's problem with the situation was that she had been accustomed to living in a city. Her mother lived on a small farm on a country road about four miles from a town of approximately 3,000 people. The community was 55 miles from the nearest large city. Probably more important, Cora saw her mother as a domineering individual. As Cora expressed it, "Those two (Lou and her mother) are so alike and they gang up on me." Although she laughed when she said this, she said it with a great deal of emotion.

Then, about six months after the move, Lou had his stroke. Cora said she felt "completely devastated and alone." She thought that part of her distress was from her heart condition. She felt quite limited by her own health and then was faced with the need to care for two dependent adults. She was often unable to drive and disliked having to depend on friends to transport her and Lou.

Observations of Lou as He Began Treatment

Cora's assessment of Lou's motor and verbal status was confirmed by clinical observation and testing. A year after his stroke. Lou's appearance was that of a tall, heavy-set man whose mask-like expression made him appear older than his age of 59.

When Lou was first seen for treatment, he used a wheelchair. He infrequently attempted to walk, and when he did use his walker, his movements were tentative, halting, and extremely slow. He seemed depressed and passive, although frequently his vague facial expression was broken by an angry scowl. Often his anger appeared when Cora tried to direct his behavior. On the other hand, Lou sometimes looked bewildered when being given a direction, as when a clinician asked him to sit down at a table.

In addition to his severe right hemiplegia and aphasia, Lou's speech was severely apraxic. His verbal output was confined to unintelligible syllables, none of which was accompanied by a change in facial expression. He seldom used gestures. He did not attempt to converse.

During initial testing, Lou sat for most of the time slumped forward with head bent and eyes downcast. He occasionally rubbed at his heavily braced right leg. He initiated no speech and hesitated several seconds, looking confused, before attempting to answer the clinician's questions. He did not respond verbally to her attempts at conversation, but rather, stared at her. Initial testing with the *Porch Index of Com-*

municative Ability (PICA, 1981) showed Lou's scores to be at the 36th percentile overall (graphic, 67th percentile; verbal, 11th percentile; and gestural, 36th percentile). The *Wechsler Adult Intelligence Scale* (WAIS) (Wechsler, 1955) was administered as part of neuropsychological testing. It revealed an performance IQ of 114. The neuropsychologist characterized Lou as "within the bright normal range but showing significant impairment to higher cortical functions."

Hearing acuity was found to be within normal limits through 4000 Hz, dropping to 46 dB in the right ear and to 55 dB in the left ear at 8000 Hz. During Lou's hospitalization, an audiologist had suggested trying a hearing aid on Lou's right ear to see whether this helped his auditory comprehension. Lou had subsequently purchased the aid recommended, but indicated during the initial interview that it annoyed him and he didn't wear it most of the time. Cora said Lou seemed more irritable when using the aid. Therefore the aid was removed, and clinical observations indicated there was no change in comprehension.

Cora's Conflicts

Expressing Ambivalence. During their group meetings spouses were asked to describe situations that typified interactions with their partners before and after the partners became aphasic (i.e., situations that illustrated their pre- and postaphasia communication). As participants described a situation the group leader asked them such questions as, which member of the dyad assumed the leadership role and how the person describing the situation felt about it.

Cora's description of situations in which she and Lou interacted revealed her great ambivalence about Lou and her role with him. On the one hand, Cora wanted Lou to talk. She said she prayed he would use enough verbalization that she could relate with him more like she had done prior to the stroke. On the other hand, she was enjoying the role as the dominant figure in the dyad after 30 years of feeling dominated by Lou. She wanted to play nurse and mother to him but resented terribly that she had to look after him. She was forced to make decisions she had not made before and to assume responsibilities she had not dealt with previously. She described a situation in which she was paying bills and said, "I yelled at him for not helping me but I would have yelled at him if he had tried to; I wanted to do it *myself!*" Cora's physical limitations added to her problems; a part of her longed for the days when Lou looked after her but she also felt she wanted to make decisions for herself.

When the group leader pointed out that it was important for Cora to clarify and cope with her ambivalent feelings, she blurted out angrily, and without smiling, "You bet that's right! I've been bossed *so* long, now it's my turn!" She paused, then added ruefully, "But I really can't be the boss, and I really don't want to be. I *hate* it!" And for the first time group members saw Cora cry.

Cora was helped to talk about her strong feelings so that she could better clarify her emotions and attitudes and develop strategies for coping with them. Because other group members had experienced similar feelings, they were asked to help Cora with the sorting process. Several of the group stated that they thought this project of helping Cora would help everybody.

Group members took the project of clarifying their attitudes, ideas and emotions a step further. They wanted to discuss ways they might assist their spouses to retain and build upon their existing abilities while not always letting their partners' needs take precedence over their own. Cora was smiling again as she agreed, "I need to work on that. too." Maybe I wouldn't feel so *very* angry if I felt I had a few rights, too." The clinicians in the group were learning that Cora's smiles were not always accompanied by pleasant emotions.

It seemed highly likely that Cora's past and present conflicts regarding her relationship with Lou had affected each of them and were continuing to do so. Likewise, Lou's past and present behaviors impinged upon Cora. Thus each partner probably was unwittingly intensifying the very real new problems Lou's stroke had created. It is obvious that what happened to one person in the dyad would greatly affect the other. Therefore, the story of Cora's change and development will be told in context of Lou's successes and failures in treatment.

Understanding Her Anger. As Cora expressed her ambivalent feelings about Lou she became more aware of her anger toward him. This anger was like a boil that had festered within her for a long time which, once touched, poured forth with a vengeance. In the group she cited example after example from the past and present to illustrate Lou's domineering ways, her helplessness in the face of his rage, and her resentment of the way he treated her. In fact, she often aired her anger for much of her talking time in the first weeks of her first series of group meetings. It seemed to the leader and students in the group that Cora's resentments permeated most of her group interactions; for example, as other group members recounted situations involving their spouses, Cora often asked, "Didn't that make you mad?" or "Didn't you resent that?" As was noted previously, she also expressed a need to dominate Lou in the present situation, to see him as helpless, and as she said, "to boss him." When a group member tried to point out ways Lou could be more independent, Cora snapped back at her with, "You don't know, you don't live with him." Although she laughed as she made this response, she sounded as if she resented any attempts to encourage her to let go of either her anger or her current feeling of being in control of all situations involving Lou.

The spouse group sessions involved much more than Cora's complaining, however. There were bonds that grew between participants; as one woman said, "We're really all in the same boat." They listened to each other, spoke understandingly of others' anguish and powerless feelings. They shared and received new information. All participants had their own resentments. All group members, including Cora, shared feelings of guilt. Some of their guilt was focused on what they might have done to prevent their spouses' trauma. Others, like Cora, felt guilty about not being able, as she said, "to accept this situation and to rise above it." As discussion moved from topic to topic, individuals in the group seemed to grow to trust each other and to feel safe talking about both problems and successes.

It is fairly well understood that when people feel safe to talk about their emotions and behaviors, they are often able to change both. This is what seemed to happen to Cora. As the sessions continued Cora was able to examine the possibility that her willingness to give in to Lou's ideas and wishes may have led him to feel he had to take charge because she was unable to manage things herself. When Cora first stated this proposition, which was a new idea to her, other group members agreed that she had helped set the stage for Lou to play the dominant role. Cora elaborated her insight in this way, "I played his game real well, didn't I? I just played right into his hands. Actually, I guess I forced him to act like he did." The group leader agreed with group members who said they thought both Cora and Lou contributed to the difficulties in their relationship.

The leader then asked, "Cora, why do you think you chose to play such a dependent role?" Cora, who usually answered questions fairly quickly, hesitated a long moment before she said, "I guess I thought he liked that." There was another pause before she spoke more rapidly. "I guess I thought he'd love me if I was helpless." She laughed but there were tears in her eyes. The leader said. "And you were so afraid of losing his love." Cora nodded agreement, "I didn't know how to be lovable except helpless." Other group members were silently thoughtful, several with tears brimming, then one said, "What a hard spot!" Cora nodded silently, crying. The silence was filled with the group members' somber empathy. Finally, a woman broke the silence to say, "Lord, Cora, do I know about it. What we women go through to keep our husbands!" The group, including Cora, shared in the laughter.

Cora went on to understand that her present attempts both to cater to Lou and to control him were in part a reaction to her past hurt and anger. She also saw her present protective behaviors as stemming from her fear of losing Lou altogether.

Letting Go. Toward the end of her first semester Cora was able to say that she was overprotecting Lou. She said, "You know, I'm overprotecting him and maybe slowing down his improvement." This possibility had been suggested to Cora earlier; however, having arrived at the idea on her own, she was ready to try to behave differently.

Even though committed to changing her behavior, she found it extremely difficult to do. She spoke of her compassion for Lou as he tried to improve and of her wish to rush in to help whenever she saw him beginning to get frustrated.

Cora's first breakthrough in allowing Lou to be more independent came when she stopped insisting Lou use a wheelchair, which by that time he wasn't using at the clinic. She found to her amazement that Lou managed well at home with his cane. She also reported with delight when Lou went to church with her for the first time since his stroke. She noted that with his cane Lou began to go regularly to Sunday service and to church social functions. Since she was able to get out more, this pleased her.

Next Cora encouraged Lou to go out with his friends while she stayed at home. She laughingly reported. "I didn't have to push him out, he was ready. I was as nervous as a mother whose kid is out on a first date; but I lived through it and I knew he had a good time."

Cora began to leave Lou at home alone once a week to drive his mother to town so both could have their hair done. Lou seemed to enjoy having some time alone and Cora became less nervous about going.

It was harder for Cora to leave Lou at home with his mother so that she could go out alone. With the group's encouragement, however, she finally tested the proposition that the two disabled people could get along without her for a period of time. She told the group about her first attempt, "I stayed away a whole hour!" The group leader said, "Good for you! You did it, you lived through it and so did they. How do you feel about that?" Cora answered, "I was scared that if they got along okay, I'd feel like I wasn't needed. But Lou was so glad to see me, I decided I'd do it again." She began to spend longer times away from Lou and his mother. She rejoiced in her greater sense of freedom and sensed that Lou appreciated her trust in him by his displays of affection when she returned.

THE COURSE OF LOU'S TREATMENT

Year One

During each semester clients attend the university speech and hearing center's aphasia program, emphasis is placed both upon improving language comprehension and improving functional use of language and speech. To this end, treatment is provided for three hours per day four days a week throughout the semester. This treatment includes daily individual and small group activities in which each client works on those aspects of language in which he or she is found to be deficient. Each day there is also a time in which the entire group of clients and clinicians meet together for activities geared to social interaction. In this social group clients' birthdays and wedding anniversaries are celebrated, as are various holidays. In the absence of such causes for celebration, clinicians lead clients in activities that require motor responses as well as communication, activities such as games, making coffee, or distributing popcorn.

This social time was considered a vital part of Lou's treatment. It was hoped that such group interaction would help him reduce his great frustration and anger. However, Lou was a dour onlooker during this time. Often he sat with head bowed, not watching the action. While his clinician would encourage him to participate, he often waved her off angrily. During his first semester, Lou was not observed to smile during the social hour.

Several speech-language goals were set for Lou at the beginning of his first semester of treatment. The first goal was to improve auditory comprehension. Also, it was considered important to help Lou reduce his apraxic errors, and improve his reading comprehension in order to assist him to find a means for occupying his leisure time. During the second semester of treatment these language and speech goals remained essentially the same.

After a year of treatment Lou showed slight improvement in all language modalities, but continued to present severe apraxia. Repeated testing with the PICA showed no significant improvement in Lou's scores. Clinical observation led to the following inferences: First, there was a dramatic increase in Lou's desire to communicate in a positive fashion as evidenced by his increased initiation of communication with clinicians and with other clients. Second, although his PICA gestural scores did not reveal a marked change, he was observed to employ increased gestures in communicative interactions. Furthermore, the gestures he did use were refined and appropriate. Whereas earlier the few gestures Lou did use were inappropriate to the topic, by the end of the year it was judged that 70% to 80% of Lou's spontaneous gestures were accurate and were of considerable aid to communication.

Equally important, Lou seemed generally less depressed. He smiled often and attempted to participate in the social group. He seemed increasingly well liked by other clients, even by those who had tended to overlook him in his withdrawn phase.

During the year Lou completely abandoned his wheelchair. He used a cane with a four-pronged base. While he walked slowly, he moved with greater confidence, his gait was more rhythmic, and he could walk greater distances.

Lou reached another milestone during the summer. He decided he was fit to drive his car. He told no one except an appalled Cora of his determination to drive. Cora, trying to enlist aid in preventing what she was sure would be a tragedy, insisted Lou get approval from his neurosurgeon. To Cora's dismay and Lou's delight, the doctor approved. Cora said she finally gulped and told Lou, "Okay, go on." After several days of practice on country roads, Lou drove himself and Cora the 55 miles by interstate to the speech and hearing center. When he parked the car, he let Cora know he wanted her to go into the center first and call his clinician to the door. With the clinician staring in amazement, Lou slowly heaved his bulky body out of the car. He walked into the building, a slow but ramrod-straight individual, his face split with the widest of his smiles and his eyes twinkling, saying his version of "Surprise!" Later a clinician asked what modifications had been made to the car to accommodate Lou. He said vehemently and clearly, "Hell, no," meaning the car had not been changed. From that day on, Lou drove himself and Cora back and forth to the clinic.

Perhaps the greatest test of Cora's willingness to grant Lou greater independence came with his decision to resume driving alone. She reported how she had fought the idea. After she gave in she told the group what she had thought: "I say I want him to be more normal, so what am I doing by trying to hold him back? But I tell you, I bit off every fingernail the first time he drove to town. It was all I could do not to call the barbershop to see if he'd gotten there. I have *never* been so glad to see him come rolling home. And he was so proud, he was all smiles and hugs for me."

On the first day Lou drove them to the clinic, Cora told the group about the event and her reactions. She said, amid the group's laughter, "I was a wreck and didn't know how to handle it without worrying Lou. So I put my head back and went to sleep." Cora slept through six or eight round trips before getting comfortable enough to chat with Lou on the road. She later reported, "I'm glad I licked that fear thing because driving is really our best time alone and I think Lou enjoys the time as much as I do."

Lou reveled in his greater independence. He drove into the nearby town for haircuts or simply to communicate with the retired men who congregated at the barbershop. Lou's ability to drive was a boon because he now had something to do when he became bored, which was often. He tired easily of watching television and while his reading comprehension had improved, he was not sufficiently skillful to enjoy reading for any length of time.

Year Two

As Lou began his second year of treatment he was again given the PICA. Although he seemed less resistant to the testing than on previous occasions, his scores had improved only slightly.

Lou's case was staffed by speech-language clinicians, the staff neuropsychologist, and the leader of the spouse group. The report of Lou's neurosurgeon was also available for the staffing. It stated that Lou's physical condition was stable. At this meeting it was decided to place less emphasis in treatment on trying to develop Lou's oral expression. Rather, emphasis would be placed upon supplementing Lou's speech and gestures with a communication aid. The instrument chosen was the Sharp Memowriter.

At first Lou seemed confused about the purpose of the Memowriter. However, as he got the idea of how to use it with his left hand and saw how it helped him communicate, he was delighted.

Cora had begun to feel extremely proud of Lou's determination and his successes. Whereas early she had talked at length about her negative feelings, during the second year Cora proudly gave the spouse group example after example of Lou's improved performance. Thus, in context of acknowledging Lou's successes she was particularly devastated when clinicians at the center decided to test Lou with the communication aid. Cora sobbed as she said, "I so hoped he'd talk better. Oh, how I wanted him to talk to me again. He's tried so hard, I've tried so hard to help him. I've failed." The group leader and others spoke compassionately of her feelings of disappointment, then someone asked, "Why is it failure if this (aid) helps you understand him better?" Cora couldn't answer; and for three sessions when the question was asked, Cora said. "I'm thinking about it." Cora also reported that she was so resistant to the aid that she was totally unable to help him use it at home. Finally, Cora entered the group room one day saying, "I know why I feel like a failure. I know how to talk so I could help Lou do that; I don't know how to use the darn machine." Having figured out the problem, Cora learned how to help Lou use the Memowriter and they consistently practiced using it at home.

The Changing Relationship Between Cora and Lou. As is typical of spouses Cora still grieved for the person who formerly talked so well, and from time to time she spoke of her grief. Her feeling of loss was mitigated, however, by her elation with how much easier it was to communicate with Lou when he used the Memowriter. She also respected Lou's willingness to use the aid and his ability to do so. In fact, in the second year of their work at the clinic all those who knew Cora and Lou in the setting thought Cora consistently showed greater respect for Lou and greater appreciation of him. This inference was confirmed the day Cora said thoughtfully to the spouse group, "You know, after 30 years of marriage I think I have learned to love my husband."

Lou for his part consistently showed great fondness for Cora. In the second year he seldom expressed anger toward her while at the clinic, often smiled at her, and waved to her with a smile as he went to his treatment room. Perhaps the greatest evidence of Lou's affection was reported by Cora. She entered the first spouse group meeting after the Christmas break saying, "I can't wait to tell you all what Lou did. You all sit down quick so you can listen; this is a first." When group members became as attentive as she seemed to need, she blurted. "For the first time in our lives Lou picked out my Christmas present!" None of the other spouses looked surprised that a husband would do that. Cora continued, "You don't understand. Lou *never* chose a present for me. He sent his secretary to do it. Or when the children got older he told them to do it." As group members expressed understanding for the importance of this act to Cora, she went on tearfully, "That man drove himself to town and shopped for two hours till he found this pendant." She laughed through her tears. "He let me understand he did it himself, including the wrapping. I already knew he wrapped it from the way it looked, crooked, but so great." The group agreed Lou had good taste in jewelry and Cora said, "Yes, he does, and it's *so* beautiful to me for *so* many reasons."

During the year Lou's clinic schedule again involved individual and small group treatment and the social hour. Lou's clinician used the individual time to train Lou with the Memowriter. He learned the typing task with dogged enjoyment, first typing "yes" and "no" and then other single words. In approximately six weeks he was typing four to six word sentences, some of which were quite telegraphic but communicative.

Lou began to employ a combination of verbalization and typing complemented by gestures in all clinical situations. For example, he initiated comminication in the social hour by waving or saying "Hey" in a loud voice and pointing to the Memowriter to get attention before typing a sentence. Although Lou's form of communication was cumbersome, it enabled him to express numerous ideas, to ask questions, and to converse.

As the year progressed, so did Lou's communicative ability. Furthermore, he was more socially active while in the speech and hearing center and became close friends with two other male aphasic clients.

Although not completely free of bouts of depression and anger, for the most part he appeared happier and more relaxed. He teased Cora, other clients, and clinicians. He told jokes and sometimes saw humor in incongruous situations. Equally as important, he seemed genuinely pleased with his progress and was eager to communicate.

As the second year ended Cora was happy with Lou's progress. She felt considerable satisfaction in her role of helping him while not trying to control him. Cora also was well aware of Lou's continuing physical and communicative limitations and of her own physical problems. She summed it up as, "I think we can go it on our own now. Neither one of us is well but we sure are better and we sure are more peaceful."

When Lou was given the PICA again after his second year of treatment, his scores had changed little except on the gestural subtests. He scored overall, 43% (a 7% gain); graphic, 69% (a 2% gain); verbal, 16% (a 5% gain); and gestural, 58% (a 22% gain).

As was routine at the end of each semester of therapy, Lou's clinician met with him and Cora to detail her perceptions of his progress and to make recommendations. The clinician reviewed his PICA scores and said they revealed some progress on the gestural subtests but indicated he had reached a plateau in other speech/language abilities. He impatiently brushed off the numbers, interrupted her, nodded, and wrote. "I better." meaning "I'm better." Then he changed it to, "I good." When Cora and the clinician laughed, Lou joined them.

At the end of the conference the clinician said she felt Lou would practice at home with the Memowriter and would continue to use improved communication. She then recommended that Lou should be dismissed from the clinic with the understanding that he could return at any time he wanted more speech-language work. She asked Lou and Cora for their reactions to the recommendation. Both partners had tears in their eyes as Lou smiled and Cora laughed a joyous laugh. Lou waved his left fist in the air as if in a victory salute as he yelled, "Good, good!" Cora expressed their feelings more elaborately: "We had so hoped for this day but were afraid to count on it. We're both so tired but so much happier." Lou smiled as he reached over and fondly patted Cora's hand.

Going Forward

As Cora and Lou left the clinic for the last time a few days after the final conference, Lou shook hands with all clients and clinicians, smiling broadly as he did. Cora tearfully hugged the aphasic clients, clinicians, the clinic receptionist, and all other spouse group members.

As Lou and Cora walked slowly out to their car, another aphasic client said, "He can't talk good, but he got to be a nice guy." And a spouse group member said, "Yep, and she's a great lady, too." Perhaps these people were summarizing the general feeling that the couple's lives would be marked by both satisfactions and sorrows, but that both were better able than they had been to cope with what came to them.

REFERENCES

Chwat, S., & Gurland, G. (1981). Comparative family perspectives on aphasia: Diagnostic, treatment and counseling implications. In R. Brookshire (Ed.), *Clinical Aphasiology Conference Proceedings*. Minneapolis: BRK Publishers.

Davis, G. (1983). *A survey of adult aphasia*. Englewood Cliffs. NJ: Prentice-Hall.

Linebaugh, C., & Young-Charles, H. (1978). The counseling needs of the families of aphasic patients. In R. Brookshire (Ed.), *Clinical Aphasiology Conference Proceedings*. Minneapolis: BRK Publishers.

Newhoff, M., & Davis. G. (1978). A spouse intervention program: Planning, implementation and problems of evaluation. In R. Brookshire (Ed.), *Clinical Aphasiology Conference Proceedings*. Minneapolis: BRK Publishers.

Porch, B. (1981). *Porch Index of Communicative Ability*. (3rd Ed.). Palo Alto, CA: Consulting Psychologists Press.

Webster, E., & Newhoff, M. (1981). Intervention with families of communicative impaired adults. New York: Grune and Stratton.

Webster, E., Dans, J., & Sanders, P. (1982). Descriptions of husband wife communication pre and postaphasia. In R. Brookshire (Ed.), *Clinical Apphasiology Conference Proceedings*. Minneapolis: BRK Publishers.

Wechsler, D. (1955). *Wechsler Adult Intelligence Scale*. San Antonio: Psychological Corporation.

CHAPTER 5

Response to Treatment: A Case of Chronic Aphasia

Robert T. Wertz

> Wertz describes the response to treatment of a 49-year-old man who lived with his aphasic residuals for seven years, then reentered treatment. The patient made substantial gains on all speech and language measures and after two years of this chronic-state treatment, decided he wanted to return to work. With his persistence and some innovative treatment planning by the author, he did. Wertz's report highlights the value of treating chronic state aphasia, particularly when this treatment has functional consequences.
>
> 1. Summarize the literature reviewed by Wertz with regard to prognosis. What does this information tell us about treating chronic aphasia? What factors prompted the patient (W.G.) to seek treatment seven years after becoming aphasic?
> 2. What sorts of referrals were made by the author as he responded to the patient's question, "Do you think I can go back to work?" How did this information assist in planning treatment?
> 3. What problems were encountered by W.G. as he sought to go back to work? How were these managed by Wertz? Would this patient's aphasic deficits affect his job performance? Why or why not?

INTRODUCTION

Life provides us with platitudes that indicate sooner is better than later. Do it now! Never put off until tomorrow what can be done today. Strike while the iron is hot. While the empirical evidence supporting these maxims may be questioned, clinicians who treat aphasic patients have heeded this advice and applied it to prognosis.

Of the many variables believed to influence an aphasic patient's potential for improving language, time postonset is considered one of the most potent. Butfield and Zangwill (1946) observed less improvement in patients who began treatment after six months postonset. Wepman (1951) noted less improvement in patients who entered treatment after a year postonset. Similar results were obtained by Sands, Sarno, and Shankweiler (1969); Marshall, Tompkins, and Phillips (1982); and Pickersgill and Lincoln (1983). The first Veterans Administration Cooperative Study on Aphasia (Wertz et al., 1981) demonstrated that over 60% of aphasic patients' total improvement present at one year postonset occurs within the first three months. Treatment study data from Deal and Deal (1978), Basso, Capitani, and Vignolo (1979); and Wertz (1983) indicate that patients who enter treatment before two months postonset make more gains than patients treated later.

The evidence listed above forecasts a bleak future for the aphasic patient who does not begin treatment early postonset. Is there any sense in investing time in treatment after aphasia has become chronic? Sarno, Silverman, and Sands' (1970) results suggest there is not. Their sample of treated severe, chronic aphasic patients, an average of 27 months postonset, failed to make significantly more improvement than their chronic group of untreated patients. Conversely, Smith (1972); Broida (1977); and Aten, Caligiuri, and Holland (1982) reported significant improvement in chronic aphasic patients who received treatment after one to six years postonset. And, there is an occasional report on a single patient like Warren and Datta's (1981) who improved markedly in treatment offered over four years after he sustained brain injury. Darley (1975) concludes that treatment initiated after six months postonset results in significant improvement if the treatment is intense and extends for several months. So, do chronic aphasic patients profit from treatment? Apparently some do, and some do not.

Ability to predict an aphasic patient's future is poor (Wertz, 1978). Typically, biographic (age and time postonset), medical, (location and size of the lesion), and behavioral (severity of aphasia) variables are used to predict whether and how much improvement will occur. A second method is to employ behavioral profiles such as those provided by Schuell (1965a). Her observation of patients' initial performance on the *Minnesota Test for Differential Diagnosis of Aphasia* (Schuell, 1965b) and their subsequent improvement or the lack of it permitted the establishment of prognostic profiles that could be used with future patients. Some (Porch, Collins, and Friden, 1980; Marshall et al., 1982) have employed multiple regression analyses to produce equations designed to predict change in language. These have significant predictive precision for groups of aphasic patients, but J.L. Deal, Wertz, Kitselman, and Dwyer (1979) demonstrated their application is limited with individual patients. Finally, Wertz, LaPointe, and Rosenbek (1984) have suggested using information collected in a brief bout of prognostic treatment to determine whether continued therapy will be efficacious. They believe a patient's ability to learn, to generalize improvement on treated material to untreated material, and willingness to practice forecast a future filled with continued gains. But, none of the methods permits more than a reasonable guess about the patient's communicative future. Usually, this is expressed by an adjective—poor, guarded, fair, good.

Most clinicians are pessimistic about the probability of changing chronic aphasia, and the conflicting results reported by those who have tried make many reluctant to offer treatment to chronic aphasic patients. But at times, we do. A report on one of our efforts follows. It is an account of treating an aphasic patient who had been aphasic for over seven years, received two years of treatment in our clinic, and returned to work.

THE CASE: W.G.

W.G.'s onset of aphasia resulted from a left-hemisphere thromboembolic infarct involving the frontal-parietal-temporal lobes in February 1966 shortly after his 41st birthday. He had graduated from high school and worked his way to district manager for an oil and gas company. At onset, W.G. lived at home with his wife and two teenage children.

A chronology of W.G.'s life after onset is listed in Table 5.1. During the first year postonset, he received treatment three times a week in a university hospital speech clinic. At one year postonset, he moved west and was treated twice a week for five months in a university speech and hearing program. W.G. and his family returned to the Midwest, and he began a seven-year period of no treatment. His days were filled with volunteer work in the Veterans Administration Medical Center: gardening, fishing, and making crafts destined for sale in a vocational rehabilitation retail outlet. When we opened a speech pathology service in the VA Medical Center in 1974, he was waiting for us.

We knew the literature that predicted a small improvement in chronic aphasic patients, and we were not accustomed to enrolling them

TABLE 5.1
W. G.'s Chronological Data

EVENT	DATES	DURATION
Left Hemisphere CVA	2/12/66	—
Speech and Language Treatment	2/66–2/67	12 Months
Speech and Language Treatment	3/67–8/67	5 Months
No Treatment	9/67–11/74	7 Years 2 Months
Speech and Language Treatment	11/74–2/77	2 Years 3 Months
Employment	2/77–Present	—

in treatment. We frowned, but W.G. was tenacious. He asked, "What do we do first?" So, we suggested a speech and language evaluation, ready to follow this with an explanation of his strengths and weaknesses, a few suggestions about how he could compensate for his deficits, and a lot of praise for how well he was coping with his residuals. We expected he would accept this traditional approach to managing chronic aphasia that our knowledge and our experience dictated.

Speech and Language Evaluation

The *Porch Index of Communicative Ability* (PICA) (Porch, 1967) indicated Overall performance was at the 71st percentile. Modality percentiles were 60th Gestural, 69th Verbal, and 76th Graphic. The PICA "high," mean performance on W.G.'s nine best subtests, was at the 70th percentile, and the "low," mean performance on his nine poorest subtests, was at the 72nd percentile. The PICA Modality Response Summary is shown in Figure 5.1, and W.G.'s writing ability on PICA Graphic Subtest A is shown in Figure 5.2.

The minimal auditory comprehension deficits seen on the PICA auditory subtests, VI and X, increased on the *Token Test* (DeRenzi & Vignolo, 1962). Performance was 15 correct on the 61 item test, and placed him at the 60th percentile for aphasic patients. Word-finding deficits were apparent on the *Word Fluency Measure* (Borkowski, Benton, & Spreen, 1967), 12 words produced and 20th percentile performance, belying W.G.'s relatively intact naming on PICA subtest IV. His score on the *Coloured Progressive Matrices* (Raven, 1962) was 27 correct on the 36 item test, placing him at the 60th percentile. Finally, a motor speech evaluation revealed no dysarthria, but a mild apraxia of speech was present. W.G. displayed a few sound substitutions in multisyllabic word repetition, initiation difficulties, and abnormal prosody. If we had classified his aphasia, the appropriate adjective would have

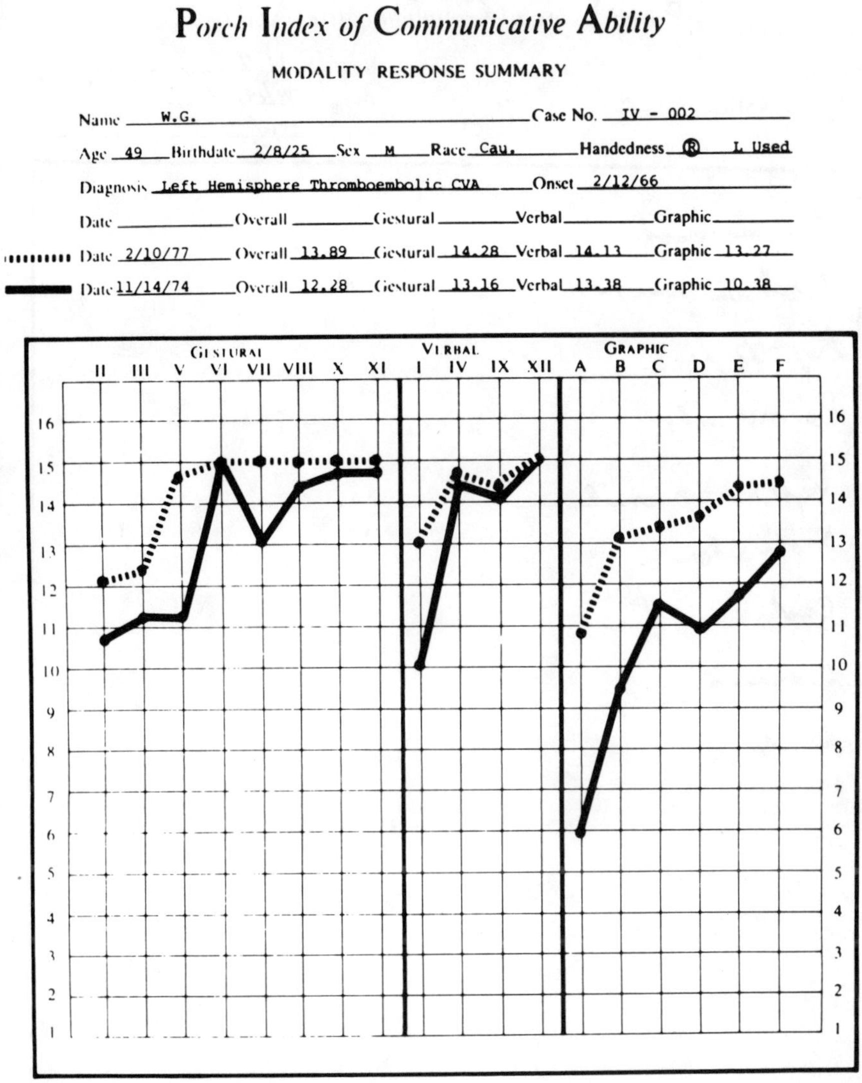

Porch Index of Communicative Ability

MODALITY RESPONSE SUMMARY

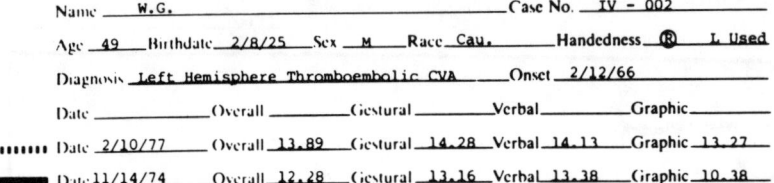

Name __W.G._____ Case No. __IV - 002__

Age __49__ Birthdate __2/8/25__ Sex __M__ Race __Cau.__ Handedness __Ⓡ__ L Used

Diagnosis __Left Hemisphere Thromboembolic CVA__ Onset __2/12/66__

Date _____ Overall _____ Gestural _____ Verbal _____ Graphic _____

••••••• Date __2/10/77__ Overall __13.89__ Gestural __14.28__ Verbal __14.13__ Graphic __13.27__

▬▬▬ Date __11/14/74__ Overall __12.28__ Gestural __13.16__ Verbal __13.38__ Graphic __10.38__

Figure 5.1 PICA Modality Response Summary showing W.G.'s pre- and post-treatment performance.

been Broca's. The speech and language evaluation results are summarized in Table 5.2.

We summarized the evaluation data in a general statement: "Patient displays a moderate aphasia crossing all communicative modalities coexisting with a mild apraxia of speech." As always, stating a prognosis was difficult. Positive prognostic signs were his age, 49; etiology,

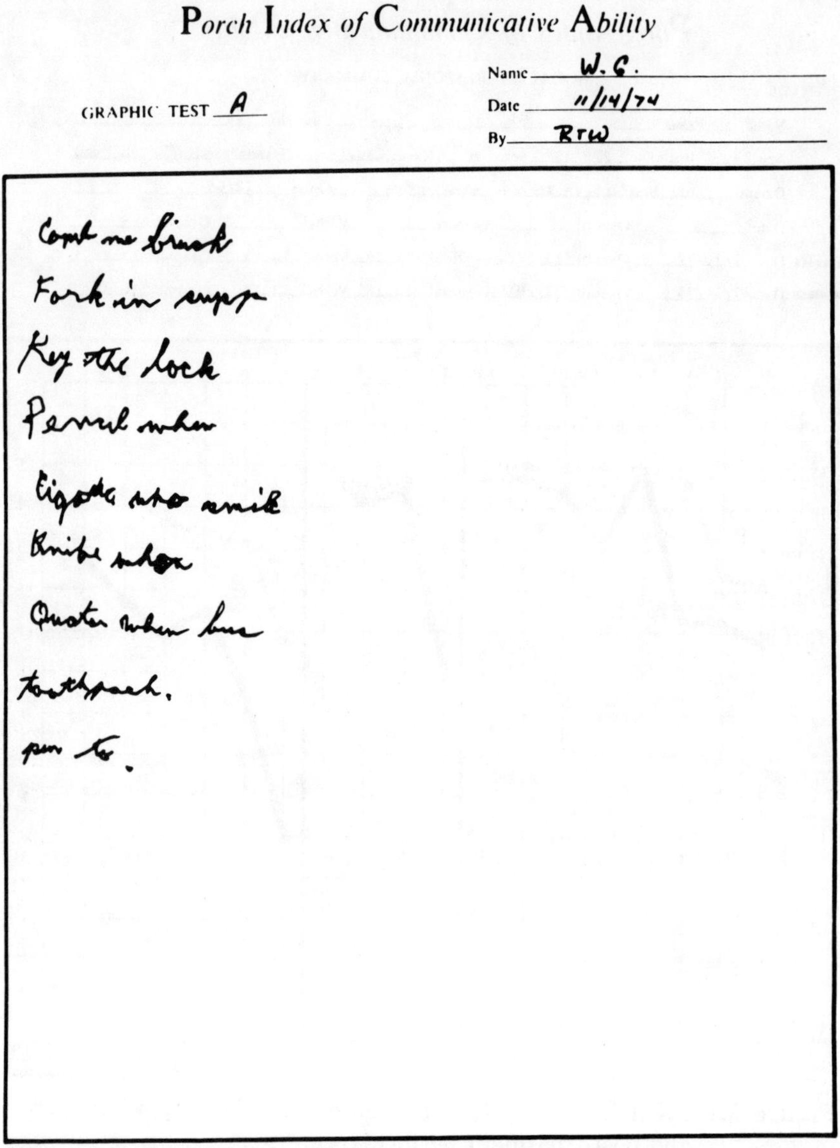
Porch Index of Communicative Ability

GRAPHIC TEST A

Name W. G.

Date 11/14/74

By RTW

Comb me brush

Fork in supp

Key the lock

Pencil when

Cigarette who smik

Knife whon

Quarter when bus

toothpach.

pen to.

Figure 5.2 W.G.'s performance on PICA Graphic Subtest A, writing the function of objects, pretreatment.

a single left hemisphere thromboembolic infarct; and severity of aphasia, moderate. Conversely, there was no significant PICA "high-low" gap to close; auditory comprehension for lengthy and complex stimuli was poor; ability to develop and use a strategy to generate words on the Word

TABLE 5.2
Evaluation Results Pretreatment

MEASURE	SCORE	PERCENTILE
PICA		
Overall	12.28	71st
Gestural	13.16	60th
Verbal	13.38	69th
Graphic	10.38	76th
Token Test	15/61	60th
Word Fluency Measure	12	20th
Coloured Progressive Matrices	27/36	60th

Fluency Measure was absent; and, most important, W.G. was almost nine years postonset. We wrote: "Patient's duration of aphasia indicates a poor prognosis for significant change in language."

Using all we had learned from the literature, our collective experience, and the results of our evaluation, we made an irrational decision and accepted W.G. for treatment. Why? Certainly we could not support electing to treat with a mass of unfavorable evidence. We answered, "Chronic aphasic patients do not improve," with, "How do we *know* that?" The literature, at that time, did not build an irrefutable case for or against treating chronic aphasia. Also, there was something about W.G. that indicated he was ready to try. The ambience of the evaluation room was upbeat. He worked hard to show us what he could do and what he could not. Finally, and most important, we could not talk him out of trying treatment. So, we said, "Patient will be enrolled in a brief period of trial treatment to reduce his chronic-state behavior and to develop some compensatory strategies for coping with his residuals." Our prose was as ambiguous as we could make it, and we hoped it would be unintelligible to most who read it. The "trial treatment" lasted for two years and three months. W.G. knew something we did not.

Treatment

Many believe that patients who have been aphasic for a long time develop "chronic state" behaviors. These behaviors are viewed as maladaptive, because they interfere with the patient's potential to communicate. They range from attempting to answer when the question has not been understood to not responding when one is able to. Treatment to eliminate chronic state behaviors begins with listing what the patient does that he should not and what the patient does not do that he should do. This procedure is followed by replacing what interferes with what is productive. For example, the patient who responds without having understood what was said can be encouraged to request a repetition, "Ah, say it again." The patient who does not respond when he might is encouraged to try by utilizing a variety of modes—gesturing, writing, drawing—and not just speaking.

Surprisingly, W.G. displayed no chronic state behaviors that seriously eroded his ability to communicate. So, our initial efforts were guided by what he wanted to change and what we thought might be possible. The approach was piebald; characterized more by tradition and inertia than by creativity. It was offered in one-hour sessions three days a week.

The treatment goals in each modality, shown in Table 5.3, were accomplished with traditional techniques—pointing, gesturing, repeating, sentence completion. confrontation naming, sentence formulation, copying, writing to dictation, and spontaneous writing. Performance on drilled tasks was recorded on the early version of Base 10 Response Forms (LaPointe, 1979), and a check on the patient's functional use of the drilled material was done at the end of each treatment session. Typically, we would establish baseline performance on a specific task with a large corpus of stimuli, select a subset of these for practice, work until criterion performance was reached, and reevaluate performance with the full corpus to look for generalization from treated to untreated stimuli. This work was supplemented with homework in reading and writing and with the Language Master drill after we were convinced W.G. did not practice his mistakes at home. Thus, treatment was pretty standard fare.

TABLE 5.3
Treatment Targets and Treatment Goals

MODALITY	GOAL
Auditory Comprehension	Increase comprehension for length and complexity
Reading	Improve word recognition and sentence comprehension
Speaking	Improve word-finding and reduce agrammatism
Writing	Improve spelling and syntax

Progress

Three months' effort convinced us some of W.G.'s deficits were being ameliorated. Reevaluation with the PICA, shown in Figure 5.3, indicated overall performance had jumped to the 89th percentile, and other measures showed similar gains. Data from treatment sessions verified progress on specific tasks, and the number of these were fattening W.G.'s

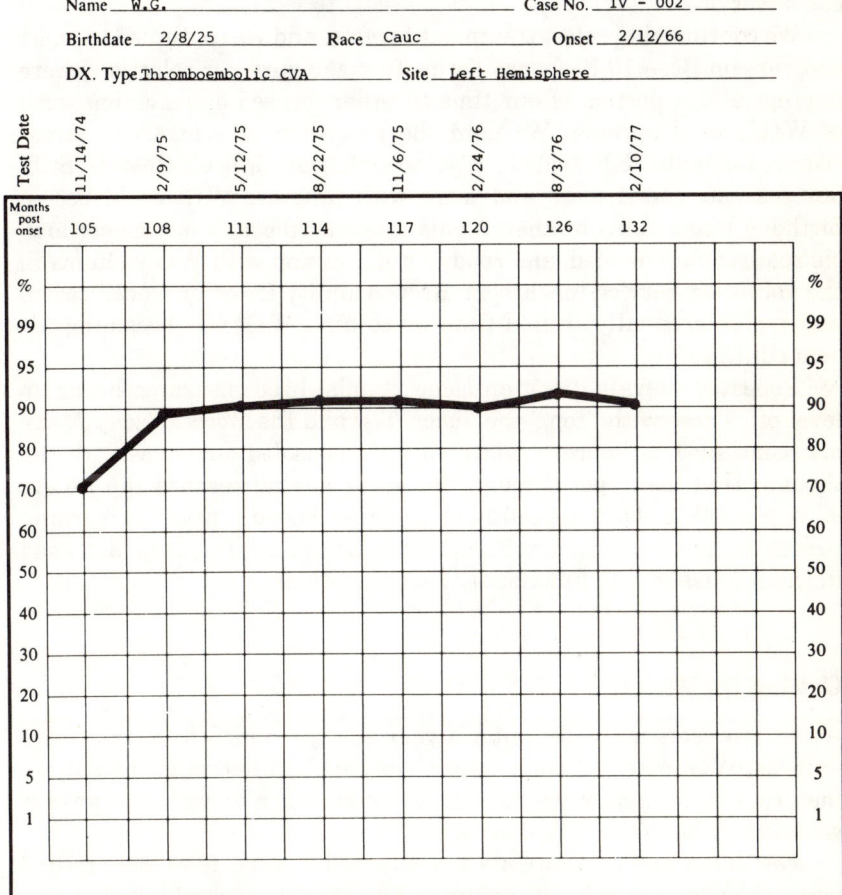

Figure 5.3 PICA Aphasia Recovery Curve showing change in W.G.'s Overall percentiles during two years and three months of treatment.

treatment folder. Comparison of baseline measures with posttreatment performance on specific tasks indicated he was learning and that gains on treated stimuli were generalizing to untreated stimuli. His willingness to practice was evident in completed homework and his desire to continue when we thought it was time for lunch. W.G. felt good about what he was doing. He should have, because he was doing well.

So, we continued. In fact, we continued for two years and three months. Treatment emphasis gradually moved to what is now called "functional," we spent more time on what people use language for and less time on those treatment tasks that supposedly get one to the point of using language. Pointing to pictures when named may improve severe auditory comprehension deficits, but it is difficult to work into a conversation.

We continued to select treatment targets, and we continued to chart progress on Base 10 Response Forms to make sure our selections were appropriate. A portion of our time together focused on resolving some of W.G.'s mild apraxia. We used the procedure of contrastive stress (Wertz, LaPointe, & Rosenbek, 1984) to drill some difficult clusters. Still, our sessions ended more and more with products W.G. could use—a birthday letter to his brother; a balanced checkbook; a newspaper article read, comprehended, and ready for discussion with W.G.'s chums in the voluntary service lunchroom. Responsibility for error identification and repair gradually shifted from us to him. W.G. was becoming his own clinician.

Repeated reevaluations on some standardized measures began to level off. Those with "top," the *Token Test* and the *Word Fluency Measure*, continued to improve minimally. We consoled ourselves with the thought that many get through life never having reached the PICA's 99th percentile. Our measures of progress became positive learning curves on Base 10 Response Forms when we reverted to unravel a snag in the line leading to functional communication.

Getting On With It

About ten years postonset, after a year and three months of treatment with us, W.G. revealed what he probably had on his mind the day we met. He asked whether we thought he could return to work. Our answer was underwhelming, "We don't know."

Few of our previous patients had returned to work. Most were retired when they became aphasic, and most had persisting residuals that precluded working as a realistic goal. We knew W.G. had progressed. He was not "normal," but, most of the time, he was functional. We wondered, functional for what?

Knowing to refer when a patient's needs extend beyond one's expertise is essential. We told W.G. that we had experienced some success in improving his language deficits, but questions about employment should be answered by someone in vocational rehabilitation. As usual, he was a couple of steps ahead of us. W.G. related he had been through vocational rehabilitation and it had ended unsuccessfully in his basement workshop constructing items for sale in a retail outlet. Crafting wooden planters and toy trucks did not meet his definition of a full-time profession. And, as usual, W.G. had done his homework. He had identified a job in our medical center that he thought he could do.

Two problems arose. First, the salary for the job W.G. was interested in was less than the income he received from disability payments. Second, he would have to pass a written examination to qualify for the job. Thus, he was faced with earning less by working than by not working, and the work he could do was a job he could not qualify for because his language skills, though improved, did not enable him to pass a written exam. Nevertheless, W.G. wanted to try. His wife was working, his son was working, and his daughter was working. He thought it was time for him to "get on with it."

At that time, W.G. performed at the 91st percentile overall on the PICA. He convinced us that a paycheck may be more fulfilling than shooting for the 92nd percentile. We obtained a copy of the examination W.G. would have to pass, and we began to tutor him.

We began by finding out which parts of the test he could pass, which needed a little work, which were within reach, and which parts were so difficult they should be ignored. Hierarchies of difficulty were constructed and W.G. was drilled. We taught him a few minor strategies in test taking; for example, how to reduce alternatives in multiple choice questions by eliminating those that that did not apply and thus increasing the probability of a correct guess. A civil service examiner was contacted, and she explained that handicapped applicants were given unlimited time and could make written or oral responses on the exam. We incorporated this information in our preparation and enacted the role of examiner for W.G., using our best bureaucratic demeanor for full effect. Three months later W.G. took the test and failed.

Persistence Is...

Taking the Civil Service examination was a great idea but a miserable reality. However, we suffered more "angst" than W.G. He inquired, "What do we do next?" Perhaps we should not have given him Eisenson's *Examining for Aphasia* (1954), because when he read, "Persistence is essential to success," he believed it. We believed the axiom, "If at first you don't succeed, try, try again," often should be paraphrased to, "If at first you don't succeed, try something else." So, we did.

A little digging disclosed that one can have certain disorders and be exempt from taking a test to qualify for U.S. Civil Service positions. Unfortunately, aphasia is not one of them. However, mental retardation is. W.G. suggested having a government vocational psychologist see if he were mentally retarded. Simultaneously, we looked for a job in our VA medical center that W.G. could do and that would pay him as much as he was receiving under disability compensation. We found one in the laundry. W.G. switched his volunteer assignment to do the work that he would do if he were employed in the job we had targeted. Eventually, W.G. was evaluated by a vocational psychologist. While W.G. was not judged mentally retarded, the psychologist agreed our patient should be exempt from taking a written test to qualify for U.S. Civil Service positions.

By the time W.G.'s certification was complete, he had demonstrated his ability to do the work in the laundry. His supervisor observed W.G. did not waste time talking. And, coincidentally, a vacancy occurred for which he qualified. W.G. walked out treatment's door into the world of work.

Wrapping It Up

When does aphasia treatment end? It ends when the patient says it should. Or, it ends when there is a viable alternative to treatment; when the patient stops being a patient and becomes a "person."

W.G. and I gathered for a final evaluation about two years and three months after we met. His PICA performance on February 10, 1977, is plotted in Figure 5.1. Writing on PICA Graphic Subtest A that morning, shown in Figure 5.4, can be compared with what he did over two years earlier (Figure 5.2). His Recovery Curve, shown in Figure 5.3, indicates PICA Overall performance was at the 91st percentile. The curve had been essentially flat for two years, but W.G.'s progress and ambition had not.

Table 5.4 shows a comparison of W.G.'s initial performance with his performance when treatment ended. He made significant gains on all measures, but these probably tell only a portion about how he got from where he was to where he is. Whether treatment was responsible for putting this man back to work, I do not know, but l think it contributed to doing so. There was a moderate aphasia and a mild apraxia of speech when we started; there still is. Some have suggested that speech treatment for aphasic patients may have only a "psychological benefit." Perhaps they are correct. Knowing and working with W.G. was psychologically beneficial to me.

Porch Index of Communicative Ability

GRAPHIC TEST __A__

Name __W. G.__
Date __2/10/77__
By __RTW__

> I smoke a cigarette
> I comb my hair.
> I eat with a fork.
> I lock door with a key.
> I eat with a knife.
> I light fire with a matches.
> I write with a pen.
> I write with a pencil.
> I spean a quarter.
> I brush my teeth ~~is~~ with a toothbrush.

Figure 5.4 W.G.'s performance on PICA Graphic Subtest A, writing the function of objects, post-treatment.

Postscript

W G. called about a year ago. He and his wife were vacationing in California. Except for Christmas cards, we had been out of touch since July,

TABLE 5.4
Pre- and Posttreatment Performance on Selected Measures

MEASURE	PERCENTILES		DIFFERENCES
	11/14/74	2/10/77	
PICA			
Overall	71st	91st	+ 20
Gestural	60th	89th	+ 29
Verbal	69th	83rd	+ 14
Graphic	76th	93rd	+ 17
Token Test	60th	90th	+ 30
Word Fluency Measure	20th	90th	+ 70
Coloured Progressive Matrices	60th	90th	+ 30

1978. I asked how things were going. He asked if I knew of any laundry service supervisor positions available, because he didn't think he could advance where he was for another year.

For a while, W.G. had stalked his future in silence. As he picked up words along the trail, his pace quickened. Sometimes, when you cannot make all of the words go right you can still go. W.G. wanted to go back to work. He did.

REFERENCES

Aten, J.L., Caligiuri, M.P., Holland, A.L. (1982). The efficacy of functional communication therapy for chronic aphasic patients. *Journal of Speech and Hearing Disorders, 47,* 93–95.

Basso, A., Capitani, E., & Vignolo, L.A. (1979). Influence of rehabilitation on language skills in aphasic patients: A controlled study. *Archives of Neurology, 36,* 190–196.

Borkowski, J.G., Benton, A.L., & Spreen, O. (1967). Word fluency and brain damage. *Neuropsychologia, 5,* 135–140.

Broida, H. (1977). Language therapy effects in long term aphasia. *Archives of Physical Medicine Rehabilitation, 58,* 248–253.

Butfield, E., & Zangwill, O. (1946). Reeducation in aphasia: A review of 70 cases. *Journal of Neurology Neurosurgery Psychiatry, 9,* 75–79.

Darley, F.L. (1975). Treatment of acquired aphasis. In W. Friendlander (Ed.), *Advances in neurology: Current review of higher nervous system dysfunction* (Vol. 7), New York: Raven Press.

Deal, J.L., & Deal, L.A. (1978). Efficacy of aphasia rehabilitation: Preliminary results. In R.H. Brookshire (Ed.), *Clinical Aphasiology Conference Proceedings.* Minneapolis: BRK Publishers.

Deal, L.A., Deal, J.L., Wertz, R.T., Kitselman, K., & Dwyer, C. (1979). Statistical prediction of change in aphasia: Clinical application of multiple regression analysis. In R.H. Brookshire (Ed.), *Clinical Aphasiology Conference Proceedings.* Minneapolis: BRK Publishers.

DeRenzi, E., & Vignolo, L.A. (1962). The Token Test: A sensitive test to detect receptive disturbances in aphasics. *Brain, 85,* 665–678.
Eisenson, J. (1954). *Examining for Aphasia.* San Antonio: The Psychological Corporation.
LaPointe. L.L. (1979). *Base 10 Response Form.* Tigard, OR: C.C. Publications.
Marshall, R.C., Tompkins, C.A., & Phillips, D.S. (1982). Improvement in treated aphasia: Examination of selected prognostic factors. *Folia Phoniatrica, 34,* 305–315.
Pickersgill, M.J., & Lincoln, N.B. (1983). Prognostic indicators and the pattern of recovery of communication in aphasic stroke patients. *Journal of Neurology Neurosurgery Psychiatry, 46,* 130–139.
Porch, B.E. (1967). *Porch Index of Communication Ability.* Palo Alto, CA: Consulting Psychologists Press.
Porch, B.E., Collins, M.J., Wertz, R.T., & Friden, T. (1980). Statistical prediction of change in aphasia. *Journal of Speech and Hearing Research, 23,* 312–322.
Raven, J.C. (1962). *Coloured Progressive Matrices.* London: Lewis.
Sands, E., Sarno, M.T., & Shankweiler, D. (1969). Long-term assessment of language function in aphasia due to stroke. *Archives of Physical Medicine Rehabilitation, 50,* 202–206.
Sarno, M.T., Silverman, M., & Sands, E. (1970). Speech therapy and language recovery in severe aphasia. *Journal of Speech and Hearing Research, 13,* 607–623.
Schuell, H. (1965a). *The Minnesota Test for Differential Diagnosis of Aphasia.* Minneapolis: University of Minnesota Press.
Schuell, H. (1965b). *Differential Diagnosis of Aphasia with the Minnesota Test.* Minneapolis: University of Minnesota Press.
Smith, A. (1972). Diagnosis, intelligence, and rehabilitation of chronic aphasics: Final report. Ann Arbor: University of Michigan, Department of Physical Medicine and Rehabilitation.
Warren, R.L., & Datta, K.D. (1981). The return of speech four and one-half years post head injury: A case report. In R.H. Brookshire (Ed.), *Clinical Aphasiology Conference Proceedings.* Minneapolis: BRK Publishers.
Wepman, J.M. (1951). *Recovery from Aphasia.* New York: Ronald Press.
Wertz, R.T. (1978). Neuropathologies of speech and language: An introduction to patient management. In D.F. Johns (Ed.), *Clinical management of neurogenic communicative disorders.* Boston: Little, Brown.
Wertz, R.T. (1983). Language intervention context and setting for the aphasic adult: When? In J. Miller, D.E. Yoder, & R. Schiefelbusch (Eds.), *Contemporary issues in language intervention.* Rockville, MD: The American Speech-Language-Hearing Association. ASHA Reports 12.
Wertz, R.T., Collins, M.J., Weiss, D., Kurtzke, J.F., et al., (1981). Veterans Administration cooperative study on aphasia: A comparison of individual and group treatment. *Journal of Speech and Hearing Research, 24,* 580–594.
Wertz, R.T., LaPointe, L.L., & Rosenbek, J.C. (1984). *Apraxia of speech in adults: The disorder and its management.* New York: Grune and Stratton.

CHAPTER 6

Aphasia Treatment: Intensive and Residential

Ann A. VanDemark

> VanDemark describes the treatment of a young aphasic client seen at the Residential Aphasia Clinic (RAC) at the University of Michigan. Her contribution illustrates the importance of duration and intensity of treatment in the management of chronic aphasic persons. More importantly the author demonstrates the value of utilizing different treatment strategies at different stages in the client's recovery course.
>
> 1. What was VanDemark's rationale for the deferring of formal testing with the client? Summarize the initial work-up of the client when he was considered as a candidate for the RAC. Why did he come to the RAC?
> 2. What do baseline scores on the PICA and Token Test indicate is occurring with the patient when he is not receiving treatment? Why might the author justify continuing treatment after the first RAC session? What was the focus of treatment during the first three RAC sessions? What changes took place during session four?
> 3. What is the philosophy of the author regarding the treatment of chronic aphasic clients? Does VanDemark consider her client's treatment a total success? Why?

INTRODUCTION

Mark was 31 years old when a left posterior communicating artery aneurysm ruptured, producing a massive subarachnoid hemorrhage, dense right hemiplegia, and severe aphasia. The incident occurred the day he was to have started a new job as a social worker in a city hospital, just two weeks after completing the requirements for his MSW. This case study describes Mark's speech and language rehabilitation, from the initial bedside visit through his return to independent living and gainful employment. Special emphasis is placed upon the role of intensive, residential speech/language treatment in the course of his recovery.

MEDICAL HISTORY

Mark was in apparently good health until May 8, 1978, when he developed a sudden severe headache, stiff neck, nausea, and vomiting. He was hospitalized. A spinal tap showed bloody cerebrospinal fluid, and carotid angiography revealed a left posterior communicating artery aneurysm. He was treated with sedation and bedrest in an attempt to control hypertension before scheduling surgery. On May 15, 1978, he experienced another episode of intracranial bleeding, following which he was unresponsive, with dense right hemiplegia and right facial weakness.

On May 22, 1978, a craniotomy was performed, and the aneurysm was clipped. The persisting neurological deficits included right hemiplegia, a seizure disorder, and aphasia. A CT scan done in August, 1981, showed marked enlargement of the left lateral ventricle, moderate enlargement of the left subarachnoid spaces, and asymmetrical (left-sided) enlargement of the third ventricle. All of these were presumed to reflect loss of substance/atrophy in the left cerebral hemisphere.

SPEECH AND LANGUAGE

In the Hospital

A speech pathologist first saw Mark at bedside on May 30, 1978. After informal observation, Mark was described as having "severe reduction in auditory comprehension, reading comprehension, verbal expression and writing complicated by apraxia of speech, visual perceptual involvement, and motor planning problems." Some automatic speech could be elicited.

Initial treatment tasks included matching objects-to-objects and pictures-to-objects, tracing and copying geometric forms and alphabet letters, recognizing and imitating single words, and following one-stage commands. Formal assessment of Mark's speech and language skills was deferred until approximately 1½ months after surgery. At that time, he achieved an overall mean score of 7.26 on the *Porch Index of Communicative Abilities* (PICA) (Porch, 1967), corresponding to a 20th percentile rank.

Mark continued to receive daily speech and language treatment throughout his three-month hospitalization, and as an outpatient over the subsequent eight months.

Outpatient Treatment

Mark made consistent progress in regaining speech and language skills. His PICA Overall percentile improved from the 20th percentile in July 1978 to the 74th percentile in May 1979. Progress was steady, and reflected gains in all language modalities. At one year postonset, he still showed a wide range of scores within individual PICA subtests and a large difference between his best and poorest communicative skills, suggesting potential for further recovery (Porch, 1981). Speech and language work was temporarily discontinued at this time because Mark was enrolled in a four-week evaluation program through the Bureau of Vocational Rehabilitation. He showed a high level of motivation and determination to return to independent living and to return to work.

Mark resumed outpatient treatment in October 1979. He had been hired as a food service worker in a hospital, but had left the job because he found it boring. He expressed a wish to continue to improve his communication so as to be able to return to a social work-related field. In the words of his clinician, "Mark refuses to accept as an ending point in his rehabilitation anything less than a position which utilizes his maximum potential." Mark was seen weekly as an outpatient until April 1980. The clinician's report indicates that his progress had slowed considerably; his PICA Overall percentile remained in the low 70s. Mark was advised that his overall level of language recovery was probably close to maximum, and that he should now concentrate on "life adjustment." Characteristically, Mark refused to accept this opinion and began investigating other treatment possibilities.

Intensive, Residential Treatment

It was at this point in his rehabilitation that Mark applied for admission to the University of Michigan's Residential Aphasia Clinic (RAC). In the RAC, twelve to fourteen aphasic clients live in a dormitory facility that is part of the RAC. Clients participate in five hours of individual and group speech and language treatment per day and have "homework" assignments as well. RAC sessions last for ten weeks. Clients must be ambulatory and able to manage the activities of daily living independently. In addition to formal treatment sessions, activities are assigned to facilitate communicative interaction among the clients and to assist them in practicing newly-regained communication skills outside the clinic. Meals are served "family style," and group social events are planned. Many of the clients become active participants in the local stroke club. Typically, one or more of the clients, assisted by the clinic staff, takes on the role of social leader, and organizes parties, attendance at campus activities, and so forth.

Entry into the RAC is preceded by a comprehensive, two-day evaluation, which includes an extensive battery of speech and language tests, a social work assessment, and a neuropsychological examination. The purpose of this evaluation is to assess the potential for further speech and language recovery, to gain a picture of the client as a communicator, and to determine whether the intensive rehabilitation program and group living situations are appropriate for the individual.

Mark came for evaluation in November 1980, two and one-half years after the onset of his aphasia.

Evaluation Data

Mark's initial evaluation confirmed his already-substantial recovery of speech and language skills. He scored at the 82nd percentile overall on the PICA and was rated "3" on the severity scale of the *Boston Diagnostic Aphasia Examination* (BDAE) (Goodglass & Kaplan, 1972). He achieved 73% accuracy on the *Reading Comprehension Battery for Aphasia* (RCBA) (LaPointe & Horner, 1979) and 52% accuracy on the *Token Test* (Spreen & Benton, 1977). More specifically, Mark's auditory comprehension scores showed high accuracy for single words, but performance deteriorated rapidly as the length and complexity of the stimuli increased. Mark responded correctly to 8 of 15 commands and 7 of 12 complex items on the BDAE. His reading comprehension scores followed a similar pattern, with few errors on single words and increased difficulty with longer, more complex items. Nearly all of the errors on the RCBA occurred on inferential paragraph and morpho-syntactic reading skill.

Test scores indicated that Mark could perform all of the tasks designed to measure verbal and nonverbal agility on the BDAE; however, his performance was somewhat slow, and occasional searching and sequencing difficulties were noted. Mark could repeat single words, but his attempts to repeat phrases and sentences were characterized by word order changes, literal and verbal paraphasias. He had difficulty recalling longer stimuli. Mark showed a high level of accuracy on confrontation naming tasks (83.3% on the BDAE and 90% on the PICA), and his infrequent errors were closely related to the target word. His naming responses were often delayed.

Mark rarely produced complete sentences, and he made numerous errors in grammar and syntax. For example, in response to the "Cookie Theft" picture (Goodglass & Kaplan, 1972), he said:

> Well, the water is drip actually dripping. It full flowing over. Other guy has a stepladder. He had a fall. Probably the window the screen. Girl will be handing a cookies. This hair is long. He's falling ground. She has cookie. But he can't do that help with the chair.

In conversation, Mark's verbal skills were described as functional for informal, social exchanges requiring brief responses. More lengthy conversational discourse was characterized by telegraphic utterances, with fragmented sentences marked by literal and verbal paraphasias. Mark followed most conversational rules but had particular difficulty with topic maintenance.

Mark wrote with his left (nonpreferred) hand. Scores on both the PICA (89th percentile) and BDAE (68 of 82 items correct) identified writing as his most accurate response modality. Primer words on the BDAE were written to dictation without error. All of the words in PICA subtest B could be retrieved, with only minor spelling errors, but on the more difficult written confrontation naming task on the BDAE Mark made both retrieval and spelling errors. Writing at the sentence level was characterized by use of single words and short word groups which lacked both semantic specificity and syntactic completeness.

A neuropsychological evaluation reflected a mixture of normal and subnormal scores, which were interpreted as representing "continuing, gradual reorganization and recovery of both language and nonlanguage functions."

Mark was accompanied by his mother when he came for his evaluation. Both he and his mother were interviewed by the social worker regarding Mark's medical, educational, employment, and family background. The social worker noted that Mark had suffered many psychosocial setbacks in addition to his communicative impairment. He was divorced and had limited contact with his seven-year-old son. After several years of study in preparation for a new job, Mark now was unable to do the work for which he had been educated. Mark had sought psychological counseling after his stroke, and when he applied for admission to the RAC, the social worker indicated that he presented himself as "fairly well adjusted." The social worker felt that Mark would be comfortable in the RAC's dormitory living situation and would be a strong contributor to group activities.

Mark was regarded as an appropriate candidate for admission to the Residential Aphasia Clinic for several reasons:

1. Several speech and language deficits could be identified which, if successfully treated, would enhance his communicative abilities.
2. His speech/language recovery had plateaued with traditional treatment.
3. There were several indicators of potential for further recovery (e.g., variability among subtest scores, intermittent performance at very high levels. and the neuropsychological evidence of continuing reorganization and recovery).
4. He was highly motivated.
5. He appeared likely to adjust to and enjoy the group activity and dormitory living.

Entry to the RAC was recommended.

First Treatment Session

Mark entered the RAC in May 1981 three years after the onset of aphasia and six months after his initial evaluation. Although Mark had been receiving outpatient treatment in his community between his evaluation and before entering the RAC, his test scores were essentially unchanged. He scored 76% on the RCBA and 52% on the *Token Test*. His PICA Overall was at the 78th percentile. Mark followed conversations when the context was broad and general, but his discourse lacked specificity and sequential order. He changed the topic frequently, and he spoke in telegraphic two-to-three-word utterances with evident word retrieval deficits.

Short term goals for Mark during his first RAC 10-week session were:

1. Increase the specificity of verbal and graphic expressions.
2. Increase awareness of errors in verbal expression.
3. Increase the use of self-cueing strategies for word-retrieval.
4. Increase the accuracy of auditory comprehension at sentence and conversational levels.
5. Increase the accuracy of reading comprehension at sentence and paragraph levels.
6. Increase the accuracy of written expression at the sentence level.

Among the speech and language tasks included in Mark's first 10-week session were those presented in Table 6.1.

Three days after entering the RAC, Mark experienced a seizure. As a result, his medication was increased and his performance decreased. It was not an auspicious beginning! However, after the seizure Mark

TABLE 6.1
Speech and Language Treatment Tasks Included in the First Ten-Week RAC Session

Auditory Comprehension

1. Listening to paragraphs of varying length and complexity and responding to wh- questions.
2. Pointing to pictures representing the prepositions "in, on, under, and beside."

Reading

3. Reading silently a paragraph of not more than 30 words, underlining the main ideas, then paraphrasing the paragraph orally.
4. Unscrambling written sentences of increasing length and complexity.

Verbal Expression

5. Rehearsing word-finding strategies, specifically: incorporating a delay before verbalization, description, and gesture.
6. Providing related words in response to a target word.
7. Describing the logical order of a sequencing task.
8. Using wh- questions to provide information about a hidden stimulus.

Writing

9. Writing noun + verb + object sentences from pictures.
10. Practicing sound and symbol association by producing a word for each grapheme.

showed substantial improvement on nearly all of the individual treatment tasks; for example, an increase from 60% to 93% accuracy on comprehension of prepositions, from 80% to 98% accuracy on unscrambling sentences, from 60% to 90% accuracy on noun + verb + object sentence writing. At the end of the first RAC session, his PICA Overall was essentially unchanged (79th percentile); however, analysis of his spontaneous speech indicated substantial increases in the use of self-cues for word retrieval and in self-correction of error responses.

Mark's motivation remained strong, and he had begun to adjust to his increased seizure medication and to show some speech and language improvement. It was recommended that he return for a second ten-week session in the RAC, which he did in the fall of 1981.

Second RAC Session

When Mark returned to the RAC in the fall, his PICA scores were unchanged from the end-of-session evaluation (77th percentile), as was his score on the *Token Test* (52%).

Treatment goals for Mark for the second 10-week session were virtually the same as those established for the first session with addition of the following tasks:
1. Increasing the specificity of verbal expression by practicing and monitoring word choice, topic relevance, and appropriate use of questions.
2. Increasing the accuracy of auditory comprehension by following verbal commands of increasing complexity.
3. Improving reading comprehension by reading silently and responding to questions about newspaper articles which were rewritten by the clinician to control vocabulary and sentence structure.
4. Writing paragraphs eight sentences in length, with logical sequencing within and between sentences.

At the end of Session II, Mark's Overall PICA score had risen to the 87th percentile. He showed his most progress in the gestural modality, reflecting improvement in auditory comprehension and reading comprehension. His RCBA score had climbed to 84% correct, and his *Token Test* score to 67% correct. Mark was able to participate in group conversations and discussions with improved accuracy in word choice and maintenance of topic.

A third RAC session was recommended, and Mark returned in the winter of 1982 for another ten weeks.

Third RAC Session

At the beginning of Session III, Mark's PICA overall had decreased slightly, to the 82nd percentile, and his *Token Test* score had dropped to 61%. Analysis of spontaneous language indicated that Mark maintained topic with 60% accuracy and used grammatically complete sentences 65% of the time. Goals for this session were:

1. Increase verbal expression of abstract concepts.
2. Increase divergent semantic processing.
3. Increase verbalization of logical decision making.
4. Increase the use of self-cueing techniques.
5. Increase reading comprehension to the level of 2–3 paragraphs.
6. Increase graphic expression to 2–3 paragraphs.

Table 6.2 provides a comparison of Mark's performance on the PICA, BDAE, *Token Test*, and RCBA at the beginning of treatment and at the end of session III. At the end of treatment, Mark's Overall PICA score had improved to the 93rd percentile. He scored 86% correct on the RCBA and 69% on the *Token Test*. In spontaneous conversation, he was 85% successful in topic maintenance and spoke in grammatically complete sentences 90% of the time.

TABLE 6.2
Pre- and Posttreatment Scores at the end of RAC Session III on the PICA, BDAE, Token Test, and the RCBA

MEASURE	PRETREATMENT	POSTTREATMENT
PICA (percentile)		
Overall	81	93
Gestural	74	95
Verbal	64	70
Graphic	89	95
BDAE (percent correct)		
Auditory comprehension	52	72
Oral expression	72	81
Reading comprehension	64	69
Writing	76	80
Token Test (percent correct)	52	69
RCBA (percent correct)	73	89

At this point, the BDAE was also readministered, in order to compare Mark's performance on all of the tests which were administered at the evaluation prior to his entry into the RAC. Pre- and post-treatment scores on the BDAE, the PICA, the *Token Test* and the RCBA are presented in Table 6.2. Changes in overall language performance are reflected in the PICA Overall percentile which was 12 points higher than at the initial evaluation. With respect to specific language modalities, the scores indicated that Mark had made the most dramatic change in auditory comprehension as measured in the *Token Test*, the auditory comprehension subtests of the BDAE, and the Gestural modality score on the PICA. Mark was clearly a much better listener by the end of session III, and this affected his performance in all of the other test modalities. Reading comprehension was modestly improved on the BDAE, from 67% to 69% correct; performance on the PICA reading subtests V and VII reflected more rapid processing of answers which were correct on the first administration of the test. However, the more comprehensive RCBA demonstrated that Mark was now able to deal with complex written material. His overall percent correct increased from 73% to 86%, and he scored 90% or better on every subtest except morpho-syntactic reading skills.

In general, Mark showed more change in receptive than in expressive modalities. Oral expression scores improved from 72% to 81% correct on the BDAE and from the 64th to the 70th percentile on the PICA. Mark continued to exhibit significant word-retrieval problems, although his grammatical and conversational skills were much improved. Written expression also showed only modest changes, from the 89th to the 95th percentile on the PICA. Mark's word-retrieval deficits were evident in his writing. He was able to produce longer and more complex written sentences, and he could sequence content more logically, but these abilities were not reflected in standardized test scores.

Mark had now begun to express concerns about his employment future and his ability to live independently. It appeared that it was time to shift away from structured language treatment and focus more on functional use of residual language in a vocationally-oriented setting. A fourth RAC session was planned for him, but with substantial changes in emphasis and format.

Fourth RAC Session

In session IV, Mark's treatment program was directed toward employment skills, specifically those associated with social work, the profession for which he had been educated. Together, the supervising clinician and the RAC social worker developed a program for Mark, with goals and tasks as follows:

1. To use social interviewing skills.
   a. Read a file and plan an interview for a prospective RAC client.
   b. Role-play the interview with the clinician.
   c. Participate in the interview with the client and clinician.
   d. Participate in orientation of prospective clients.
2. To use record keeping skills.
   a. Write summary reports of interviews and other activities.
3. To use administrative skills.
   a. Participate in RAC staff meetings.
   b. Assist in the organization and development of the local stroke club.

Mark's training as a social worker was evident in his handling of the interviews. He was extremely sensitive to the emotional needs of interviewed clients and provided a great deal of positive support. His recommendations were practical and constructive. He provided potential clients with a perspective of the program that was very helpful to the clients and their families. In interview situations, however, he had a great deal of difficulty asking direct, appropriate questions. Many of his questions were incomplete in form, or he changed the topic so abruptly that the flow of the interview was disrupted and it was difficult for the interviewee to respond. Mark's summary reports of interviews and discussions with other staff members were generally accurate in content and form but reflected reduced amounts of information. His participation in staff meetings was appropriate and goal-oriented.

Perhaps the most positive aspect of the session was Mark's role in developing the local stroke club. He was a key figure in its organization, helping to plan meetings and acting as host, and displaying his ability to function capably as an organizer and group leader.

Little change in Mark's specific linguistic skills was seen during this therapy period. However, and perhaps even more important, he acquired increased confidence in his ability to communicate and to participate in situations where group leadership was needed. It also became clear to Mark that in spite of his impressive recovery, his language abilities were not yet at a level that could support his return to full professional responsibilities as a social worker.

Mark decided to focus for a time on independent living, to seek housing and whatever employment he could find in the local community, and to continue speech and language treatment on a reduced, outpatient schedule.

An Outpatient, Again!

Mark obtained a part-time job, found an apartment, and began his experiment in independent living. He participated in speech and language treatment as an outpatient two hours per week for eight weeks in the fall of 1982 and for another six weeks in the spring of 1983. During both of these sessions the focus of treatment was divergent semantic ability. Mark engaged in a number of tasks as outlined by Chapey (1981), including the identification of similarities and differences, naming, and planning elaboration. In addition, he engaged in concept-awareness tasks, problem-solving tasks. and specific exercises for reading and writing abilities.

Evaluation of divergent semantic ability was based primarily upon Mark's scores on an oral word fluency task. This task required him to produce as many words as possible beginning with a specific letter in one minute's time. Table 6.3 presents Mark's baseline scores (October 1982) and his final scores (June 1983). The numbers speak for themselves, and their impact on Mark's word retrieval abilities was evident in his conversation. These were appropriate and productive tasks for Mark.

In the summer of 1983, Mark chose to return to his home community, to be near family and friends and to seek full-time employment.

TABLE 6.3
Scores on a Word-Fluency Task Pre- and Posttreatment During the RAC Session IV

	Easy f, t, s	Moderate r, l, n	Difficult k, j, v	TOTAL
Baseline	7	8	4	19
Posttreatment	22	17	11	50

A Final Note

Following a case like Mark's over a period of several years illustrates the diversity of treatment methods that are appropriate at different stages in the recovery process. In the early weeks, when Mark's speech/language skills were so severely impaired that formal evaluation was not attempted, the treatment focused on straightforward auditory and visual matching tasks. As Mark progressed, the length and complexity of the stimuli were increased, and the tasks expanded to include all input and output modes in contexts more nearly approximating natural language use. In the final stages of treatment, Mark was required to use his language skills as well as to improve them, and he was given opportunities to practice in "real life" situations which were relevant to his own professional interests.

Mark's rehabilitation process illustrates the introduction of intensive treatment at a point when Mark's recovery had plateaued with traditional, twice-a-week outpatient treatment. Intensive treatment in a situation where there were many opportunities to use communicative skills in a comfortable environment produced substantial improvement for Mark. When he left the RAC, Mark was a proficient communicator. Intensive treatment is appropriate at different times for different individuals, but our experience suggests that it is particularly effective for the "chronic" patient, the aphasic individual who is well past the period of spontaneous recovery (Dodaro, VanDemark, Gaughan, & Lemmer, in press).

Finally, the case illustrates the importance of continuing treatment throughout the entire recovery process. Figure 6.1 shows Mark's Overall percentiles on the PICA during his treatment in the RAC. It was

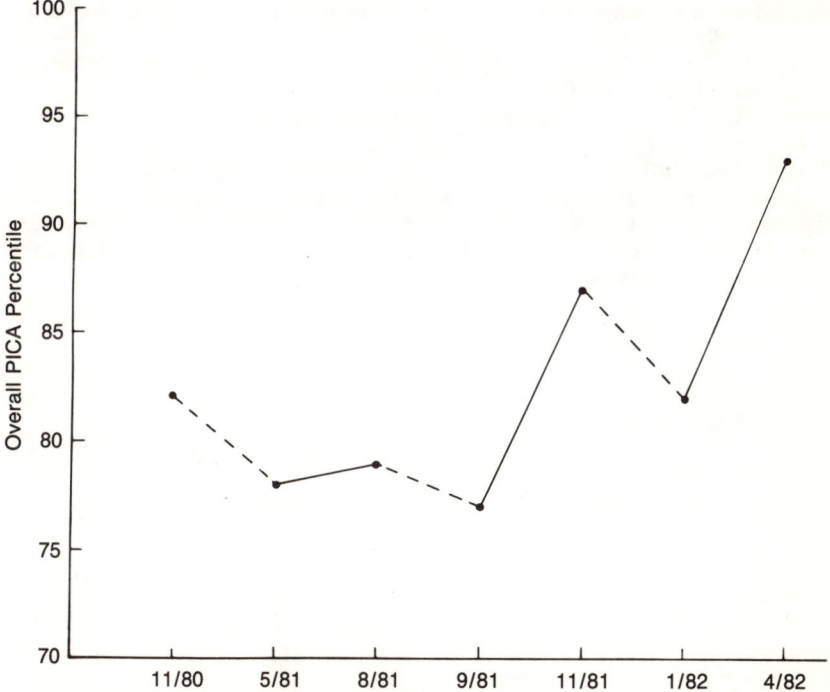

Figure 6.1 Overall PICA percentiles for Mark during treatment in the RCA. Hashed lines reflect periods when Mark did not have treatment.

typical for Mark to show an increase in his PICA Overall while he was in treatment, and to maintain or even lose a few percentile points when he was not. Reacquired language skills are fragile, and continued treatment is required to maintain them. Was Mark's treatment a success? It was and it wasn't. Six years after the onset of aphasia, Mark lives alone and manages his personal and financial affairs. He has a reasonably active social life. He holds a full-time job with a modest degree of independence and responsibility. He is satisfied for the moment, at least. But he is not able to work in the profession for which he was educated. He has come a long way back from his initial language disability, but not all the way back.

REFERENCES

Chapey, Roberta. (1981). Divergent semantic intervention. In R. Chapey (Ed.), *Language intervention strategies in adult aphasia*. Baltimore: Williams & Wilkins.
Dodaro, R., VanDemark, A., Gaughan, M., & Lemmer, E. (In press). The role of time post onset and severity in rehabilitation on chronic aphasia.
Goodglass, H., & Kaplan, E. (1972). *The assessment of aphasia and related disorders*. Philadelphia: Lea and Febiger.
LaPointe, L.L., & Horner, J. (1979). *The Reading Comprehension Battery for Aphasia*. Tigard, OR: C. C. Publications.
Porch, B.E. (1967). *Porch Index of Communicative Ability: Theory and Development* (Vol. 1). Palo Alto, CA: Consulting Psychologists Press.
Porch, B.E. (1981). *Porch Index of Communicative Ability: Theory and Development* (Vol. 2). Palo Alto, CA: Consulting Psychologists Press.
Spreen, O., & Benton, A.L. (1977). *Neurosensory Center Comprehension Examination for Aphasia*. Victoria, British Columbia: Neuropsychological Laboratory, University of Victoria.

CHAPTER 7
Maximum Recovery: By What Definition?
Sara B. Sanders

> *Sanders' chapter illustrates that standarized test results may not always be the best means of measuring maximum recovery from aphasia or determining when a patient should be discontinued from treatment. She points out the importance of being sensitive to those speech and language behaviors which the patient can improve and will have an influence on his daily life.*

1. What does Sanders mean by maximum recovery? How might this be measured? When the patient has plateaued on a specific test how can treatment results be assessed?
2. At times aphasic clients are not ready for participation in formal testing. When might this be the case? What procedures does Sanders use to obtain objective information on her client when he could not participate in formal testing?
3. Review the steps in the "verbing" program developed by Loverso, Selinger, and Prescott (1979). What types of aphasic patients is this program suited for? Why? How does Sanders document the effects of this program on the patient presented?

DETERMINING MAXIMUM RECOVERY

Aphasia clinicians use a variety of formal and informal assessment tools to determine (a) a differential diagnosis, (b) the type and severity of the patient's aphasia, (c) the presence of related deficits such as apraxia of speech, and (d) the direction treatment should take. In addition, medical (site and size of lesion), biographical (age and time postonset), and behavioral (severity of aphasia) data guide the clinician toward a reasonable decision to provide or not to provide treatment. For these reasons, the determination as to when or if an aphasic patient should be treated for a speech and/or language deficit is much easier than deciding when the patient has profited maximally from treatment.

Two serious problems confront the clinician in making a decision to terminate treatment. Premature dismissal may deprive the patient of learning additional strategies that could enhance his communication abilities. Conversely, retaining the patient in treatment too long may cause a financial burden on the family, frustrate the patient, or lead to treatment "burn out."

Textbooks that provide information on the issue of termination of aphasia treatment suggest that it should end when the patient attains maximum recovery. However, the concept of what actually constitutes maximum recovery is unclear and open to question in many individual cases. According to Davis (1983), the end of recovery is confirmed when measures of language no longer show an upward trend across time, and a plateau in language functioning is observed over a series of assessments. A common example would be an aphasic patient who showed negligible gains on a standardized test such as the *Porch Index of Communicative Ability* (PICA) (Porch, 1967) for two or three monthly testings. Unfortunately, the assessment measures employed may only reflect improvement on the areas specifically tested. Other aspects of communicative behavior may continue to have the potential for additional improvement.

The accountable aphasia clinician assesses the patient's progress in treatment continuously. Periodic administration of standardized tests such as the PICA is one way of accomplishing this, but may not be the best means of determining treatment results particularly when the speech and language behaviors stressed in the clinic are not assessed within the standardized measure. Bob, a young aphasic man seen at the Memphis Veterans Administration Medical Center (VAMC) constitutes such an example. He was provided intensive speech and language treatment until his performance showed no change on the PICA. Individual sessions were reluctantly terminated in favor of subsequent group treatment for increased socialization, but the patient continued to exhibit no improvement in his PICA scores. Ultimately, the patient requested specific assistance in improving his verbal communication. A second period of individual treatment was implemented using a "verbing" program. The patient reflected a modest gain in his PICA scores; but, more important still, he improved his functional communication to a point where he was satisfied that he had profited maximally from treatment.

THE CASE: BOB

Background Information

Bob, a 45-year-old, right-handed man, suffered a left-hemisphere cerebrovascular accident (CVA) in September 1979, six weeks after retiring from a 24-year career in the U.S. Air Force. He was a high school graduate, had attended the NCO academy, and had attained the rank of Master Sergeant. His primary service occupation was that of an airplane mechanic.

Prior to his CVA, Bob was in good health. Four months before the stroke, however, he experienced occasional episodes of tingling and weakness of the right arm and leg. Because of the intermittent nature of the symptoms, he did not seek medical attention. On the day of his stroke Bob awoke and went to the bathroom. He drank some coffee and lay down on the couch. His mother, with whom he was living at this time, noticed that he began to rub his right arm, to drool from the right side of the mouth, and could not speak. He was subsequently taken to the emergency room of the VAMC.

In the emergency room he became progressively somnolent. Neurological examination revealed that he was hemiplegic on the right and unable to look to the right side. There was no palpable edema. There was a shallow right nasolabial fold. Corneal reflexes could not be elicited on the right. There was some narrowing of the right palpebral fissure. Hyperreflexia was noted expecially with regard to biceps and knee jerk. Babinskis were elicited bilaterally with the right greater than the left. There was a positive snout reflex. Because of his deteriorating state, a cerebral angiogram was obtained. The angiogram showed a large clot in the left internal carotid artery just above its bifurcation with severely restricted filling of the left anterior circulation. There was minimal filling of the area of the left middle cerebral artery. Radioisotope brain scan revealed uptake in the left parietal area. An electroencephalogram showed polymorphic delta activities over the left hemisphere. Bob was treated with Decadron, and his mental status improved substantially. Decadron was stopped three days after admission because of the possibility of upper GI bleeding.

SPEECH AND LANGUAGE EVALUATION

Early Assessments

Bob was too ill to be brought to the clinic for evaluation immediately after his stroke. Bedside visits indicated that he had difficulty maintaining eye contact for more than a few seconds, but did attend to verbal stimuli. He looked alert and often gave the impression that he understood what was being said to him by nodding his head slightly.

At 10 days postonset the PICA was administered. As PICA testing progressed, Bob became less responsive. The Gestural and Verbal subtests were completed, but the Graphic subtests had to be terminated when Bob refused to continue. He made no verbal responses on the PICA but simply looked at the objects, then looked at the clinician, and waved his hand over the objects. On the Auditory subtests. Bob pointed incorrectly to items that were named or described. The visual matching tasks were the only subtests where he produced accurate responses. Because the PICA was not completed, an Overall score could not be computed, but Verbal and Gestural modality mean scores and percentiles were obtained. The verbal mean was 2.00 and the gestural mean was 5.94. These placed him at the 1st and 4th percentile rankings respectively in a larger random sample of left-hemisphere damaged patients (Porch, 1967).

Modified Testing. Although Bob did not respond accurately on the Auditory Comprehension subtests of the PICA, he was able to respond correctly when task demands were modified. For example, when asked to point to a picture named by the examiner in a field of three pictures, he responded correctly on 14 of 16 trials. He was also able to follow one-step commands such as "raise your hand," "wave goodbye," and "look out the window."

Although the easier PICA Graphic subtests were not completed, Bob demonstrated some residual writing ability. He copied a circle, a cross, the numbers "1, 2, 3," and his first name, with slight difficulty. However, when asked to copy his last name, he perseverated on the letter "B." He refused to copy single words.

Verbal responses could not be elicited even when Bob was provided maximum assistance through modeling and cueing, suggesting that a severe apraxia of speech coexisted with his aphasic deficits. His ability to carry out volitional movements of the oral mechanism (e.g, protrude the tongue, whistle, puff out the cheeks, etc.) was similarly impaired. He did not respond, but merely looked at the examiner.

Later Assessment

Standardized administration of the PICA at one month postonset to patients who have suffered thromboembolic insults permits the clinician to predict the patient's PICA score at six months postonset. These predictions are based on a formula that Porch (1967) calls the high-overall prediction or the HOAP slope. This computational procedure has been discussed by several writers (Wertz, L. Deal, & J. Deal, 1980; Porch and Callahan, 1981). Unfortunately, at the time his one-month PICA evaluation was scheduled, Bob developed a pulmonary embolus and could not be brought to the clinic. Reevaluation with the PICA was not carried out until October 29, 1979, six weeks after onset. By this time Bob had changed dramatically. His auditory comprehension skills improved to the point where he was able to respond accurately to most requests, providing they did not require verbal responses. He had become increasingly more independent in his self-care.

Bob's overall PICA score was at the 42nd percentile (9.81). Modality percentiles were: Gestural, 53rd percentile (12.89); Verbal, 28th percentile (5.55); and Graphic, 62nd percentile (8.53). A comparison of the verbal and gestural scores with those from the first evaluation revealed marked improvement. His verbal scores had increased by 27 percentile points, and his gestural scores had increased by 49 percentile points. His predicted overall score at six month postonset was the 75th percentile.

The most notable residual deficit at the time of reevaluation was that Bob was still nonverbal. He recognized his inability to perform voluntary movements of the oral mechanism, and he shook his head negatively when asked to respond verbally. This behavior prompted a diagnosis of "elective mutism" by two different physicians which colored the attitude of ward personnel who felt that Bob was deliberately refusing to speak. This had unfortunate consequences when Bob finally did produce his first verbalization, "I don't know." Ward personnel, family members, and physicians lavished him with positive reinforcement for this intelligible and somewhat successful verbalization and it became a stereotypic utterance.

TREATMENT

Bob's speech and language rehabilitation spanned approximately three years and is presented in four segments: (a) individual treatment concentrating on amelioration of deficits in all language modalities, (b) group treatment for increased socialization, (c) group treatment plus spouse counseling, and (d) individual treatment emphasizing improvement in verbal expression through the use of a verbing program. The PICA was administered periodically throughout each phase of treatment as a measure of treatment efficacy.

Individual Treatment

All test results indicated that Bob was severely impaired in all language modalities. Six areas were selected for treatment: auditory comprehension, oral motor sequencing and speech production, word retrieval, gestural communication, reading comprehension, and graphic skills.

Auditory Comprehension. Initial efforts to improve Bob's auditory comprehension were carried out at bedside as he was too ill to come to the clinic. These focused on recognition of familiar sounds, answering yes/no questions with head nods, following one and two step commands, and identification of objects and body parts. When he could be brought to the clinic, sentence comprehension and other more difficult tasks were introduced. Eventually his auditory comprehension improved to a point where he only had difficulty with complex stimuli.

Apraxia of Speech. Initial treatment of Bob's severe oral apraxia included manipulation of the oral mechanism and imitation of oral movements. This often involved using a mirror to stimulate him to open the mouth, protrude, lateralize, elevate the tongue, pucker the lips, smile, puff out the cheeks, vary lip pressure, and produce various vowel sounds. As oral apraxia lessened, treatment for the apraxia of speech was initiated. This involved articulatory drill focusing on appropriate placement, timing, and sequencing, beginning with the visual labial and lingual plosive sounds and moving to the more obscure velar plosives, as well as fricatives and affricatives.

Gestures. Because Bob could not communicate verbally immediately poststroke, attempts were made to establish a gestural system for communication. Bob initially responded to this treatment with obscure and imprecise gestures (even though he did not appear to have limb apraxia). His gestures eventually became more efficient but he did not use them outside the clinic. He continued to attempt to vocalize in order to communicate, even when this was unsuccessful.

Word Retrieval. Retrieval and production of single words (nouns and verbs) began with imitation tasks. When Bob could produce approximations to the clinician's models, cueing strategies were employed to elicit nonimitative production of target words. Phonemic cues consisting of the first sound of the word provided by the clinician were most successful. Bob's attempts to provide his own phonemic cues were unsuccessful. Since the intent of cueing was ultimately to have

Bob generate his own cues, and he was not stimulable for phonemic cueing on his own, semantic cues in the form of a functional associate (e.g., drive-car) were employed.

To elicit single word productions beyond an imitation level a hierarchical cuing procedure was followed. This began with the clinician providing sentence completion cues (e.g., "You read a _____"), moving to semantic cues (e.g., "You read it") and then having Bob provide his own self-cue. In cases where he could not produce a semantic cue independently, he would sometimes draw the initial letter of the word with his finger on the table or in the air. This was usually effective in facilitating production of the target word.

Accuracy criteria were set for each step of the hierarchy, and ultimately the clinician introduced tasks and provided semantic cues in a nonstructured format. The overall objective of the process was to get Bob to provide his own cues. Hence, the clinician and Bob were primarily concerned with finding the cueing stategy most effective for Bob in the word-retrieval process.

Reading Comprehension

Reading was not addressed in the early stages of recovery. However, as auditory comprehension, verbal expression, and word retrieval began to improve, reading tasks were added to the treatment repertoire. This began with the matching of single words with appropriate objects or pictures. Bob progressed to a point where he could read and comprehend simple declarative sentences. He continued to have problems understanding prepositions, subjunctives, and passive voice. Moreover, as the visual stimuli became more lengthy and more complex, Bob was unable to respond accurately.

Graphic Skills. Bob had a severe right hemiplegia and had to use his left hand for writing. He was given simple tracing tasks to improve fine motor coordination of his left hand. These tasks were followed by copying tasks (shapes, numbers, alphabet, and his name). He was subsequently asked to copy single words and then to write these same words from dictation. This activity was followed by written confrontation naming tasks. Eventually Bob could write simple sentences, but these were usually grammatically incomplete and included misspelled words.

Termination of Individual Treatment. Table 7.1 gives Bob's mean scores and percentile rankings for the PICA Overall, Gestural, Verbal, and Graphic subtests throughout 16 months of individual treatment. These data show clearly that he made steady and marked progress in all areas in the first ten months of treatment (tests 1–6), at which time he reached his predicted target percentile on the PICA. From ten to fourteen months postonset, and from fourteen to sixteen months

TABLE 7.1
Client's Overall and Modality Percentile Rankings and Scores on the *Porch Index of Communicative Ability* Throughout Thirty-nine Months of Treatment

Treatment	Test Number	MPO	Overall	Gestural	Verbal	Graphic
Individual Treatment	1	1	None	5.94 (4%)	2.00 (1%)	None
	2	1.5	9.81 (42%)	12.89 (53%)	5.55 (28%)	8.53 (52%)
	3	3	11.21 (56%)	13.01 (56%)	8.83 (41%)	10.40 (77%)
	4	5	11.99 (67%)	13.25 (63%)	10.58 (48%)	11.25 (82%)
	5	8	11.74 (64%)	12.95 (55%)	11.65 (53%)	10.20 (75%)
	6	10	12.35 (72%)	13.49 (68%)	12.08 (55%)	11.02 (81%)
	7	14	12.63 (76%)	13.60 (71%)	12.45 (58%)	11.45 (84%)
	8	16	12.57 (75%)	13.19 (61%)	12.70 (60%)	11.65 (85%)
Group Only	9	19	12.68 (77%)	13.69 (73%)	12.60 (59%)	11.38 (83%)
Group and Spouse Counsel	10	20	12.59 (75%)	13.79 (76%)	13.00 (64%)	10.72 (79%)
	11	25	12.73 (77%)	13.78 (76%)	12.95 (63%)	11.18 (82%)
	12	27	12.73 (77%)	13.81 (76%)	13.13 (65%)	11.08 (81%)
"Verbing" Program	13	29	13.02 (81%)	14.06 (82%)	13.37 (69%)	11.55 (84%)
	14	32	12.95 (80%)	13.95 (80%)	13.38 (69%)	11.33 (83%)
	15	37	13.28 (84%)	14.29 (90%)	13.28 (68%)	11.93 (87%)
	16	39	13.26 (84%)	14.27 (89%)	13.37 (69%)	11.85 (86%)

postonset, however, his PICA Overall scores reflected only modest changes, and his gestural score dropped ten percentile points in the latter interval. This leveling off in PICA performance occurred when Bob was receiving a substantial amount of treatment; hence, it was regarded as a signal that treatment should be terminated.

Group Treatment

To provide Bob some opportunity for socialization he was enrolled in a weekly aphasia group meeting. The group meeting was divided into a half hour of discussion of current events followed by a half hour of instruction in which participants worked on individual goals. Bob's goal was to increase the amount of his verbalization. Unfortunately, the subsequent PICA evaluation following three months group treatment indicated no change in his overall performance (see Table 7.1).

Spouse Counseling

Domestic problems existed in Bob's life both before and after the stroke. He had been divorced from his first wife for several years. He remarried seven years before his stroke but had separated from the second wife two weeks before the insult and gone to live with his mother. Approximately two months following his hospital discharge, his wife took Bob back home to live with her. This situation was full of turmoil and there was some question as to whether Bob's support system was optimal for promoting his most efficient communication. His wife had become increasingly assertive, making all the decisions, and had essentially alienated Bob from the four children of his first marriage. A period of spouse counseling in conjunction with Bob's continued group treatment was proposed. His wife agreed to attend a spouse group geared toward discussions of the impact of stroke on the family and to air any feelings of resentment or anger. In addition, she and Bob began attending the community stroke club where they eventually assumed a leadership role. Although Bob's PICA scores (Table 7.1) did not change after one month of group treatment and spouse counseling, he requested more individual treatment to increase his verbal communication. He seemed quite motivated to attempt anything in order to improve his verbal performance.

Bob's Input

Bob's PICA performance when he reentered individual treatment at 25 months postonset indicated no change from prior testing (see Table 7.1). However, he felt he could make additional improvement in his verbal communication. Typically, Bob spoke in short agrammatic statements consisting of a noun-verb (e.g., "fire burn") or a verb-object (e.g., "eat cake") combinations. In addition, he still had difficulty retrieving words promptly and had problems completing the articulation of multisyllabic words (e.g., "impossible") without a significant time lapse. Bob's behavior and input to the clinicians identified two communicative behaviors (short agrammatic utterances and increased latencies) that they felt, if improved, would improve his communication. Based on this input, a specific program was implemented to ameliorate these deficits.

Verbal Program. The "verbing" program (Loverso, Selinger, & Prescott, 1979) is divided into lwo levels of response. The first involves a subject-verb construction, the second a subject-verb-object construction. The program uses clinician modeling techniques and *wh* word cues (e.g., who, what, etc.) to assist the patient in generating a sentence by selecting the subject-object from a group of foils. Target responses, cue words, and groups of words from which to choose the subject or object are provided for the patient. The ultimate object of the program is to elicit these sentence forms from the patient. Table 7.2 gives examples of stimuli and expected responses.

A modification to the program was made where Bob generated his own *wh*-words as a self-cue to decrease response latency. For example, Bob was able to look at a picture, state the verb, and ask "who" to facilitate the subject response or ask "what" to facilitate the object response. At the end of the program, Bob appeared to execute these cues silently. Clinician feedback was provided by helping Bob graph his response latency times and the mean length of utterances each week.

Treatment Probes. To evaluate the effectiveness of the verbing program, baseline measures were taken over three consecutive days, and baseline probes were administered once a week throughout treatment. These involved having Bob describe action pictures, record his descriptions, and measure the length of his utterances. Response latency was defined as the time it took him to complete a specific utterance and was timed using a stopwatch. At the end of the "verbing" program, response latency was reduced from an average of 17.6 seconds during baseline to an average of 4.3 seconds per utterance (Figure 7.1). Bob's mean length of utterance increased from an average of 2.3 words at baseline to an average of 5.2 words. Figure 7.2 illustrates the increase in mean length of utterance based on the baseline and treatment probes. Examples of his responses obtained before and after the completion of the verbing program are cited below.

During Baseline Probes:
    Example 1: "... man ... leaves ... cold" (Picture of a man raking leaves in the fall.)
    Example 2: "... woman ... plate ... cup" (Picture of a woman washing dishes.)

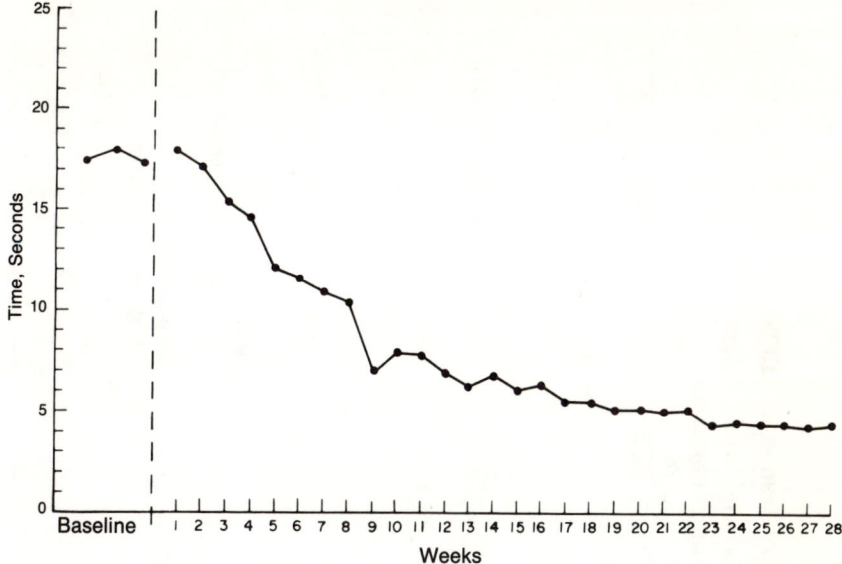

Figure 7.1 Mean length of utterance throughout "verbing" program.

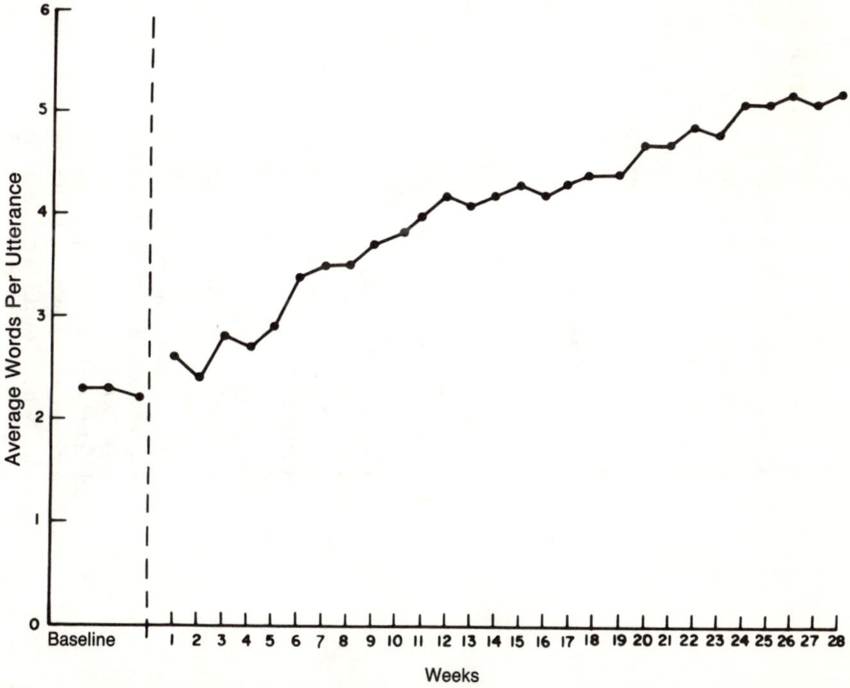

Figure 7.2 Mean response latency (in seconds) throughout "verbing" program.

TABLE 7.2
Examples of "Verbing" Program Stimuli (Loverso et al., 1979)

[Materials: 30 verb cards; 6 *wh* question cards (who, what, where, when, why, how); subject and object cards; and subject and object choice cards]

LEVEL	STIMULI	RESPONSE
I-A	Verb–graphic and verbal (e.g., "eat" written on card and shown to patient while clinician says "eat")	Repeat verb (e.g., patient repeats "eat")
	Wh cue–graphic and verbal (e.g., patient shown "who" card while clinician says "who")	Repeat *Wh* cue (e.g., patient repeats "who")
	An appropriate subject–graphic and verbal (e.g., patient shown card with "I" written on it while clinician says "I")	Repeat subject (e.g., patient repeats "I")
	S + V – graphic and verbal (e.g., clinician says "I eat" while pointing to appropriate cards)	Repeat S + V (e.g., patient repeats "I eat")
I-B	Verb–graphic and verbal (e.g., patient shown "eat" card while clinician says "eat")	Repeat verb (e.g., patient repeats "eat")
	Wh cue–graphic and verbal (e.g., patient shown "who" card while clinician says "who")	Repeat *Wh* cue (e.g., patient repeats "who")
	Subject choice card–graphic only (e.g., patient shown card with written words, "I," "who," "bird," "she," and "dog")	Choose correct subject (e.g., patient says "I")

TABLE 7.2 Continued

LEVEL	STIMULI	RESPONSE
II-B	Verb–graphic and verbal (e.g., patient shown "eat" card while clinician says "eat")	Repeat verb (e.g., patient repeats "eat")
	Wh subject cue–graphic and verbal (e.g., patient shown "who" card while clinician says "who")	Repeat Wh subject cue (e.g., patient repeats "who")
	Subject choice card–graphic only (e.g., patient shown card with words "I," "who," "bird," "she," and "dog")	Choose correct subject (e.g., patient repeats "what")
	Wh object cue–graphic and verbal (e.g., patient shown "what" card while clinician says "what")	
	Object choice card–graphic only (e.g., patient shown card with words "trees," "steak," "light," "one," and "money")	Choose correct object (e.g., patient says "steak") Generate $S + V + O$ (e.g., patient says "I eat steak")
II	Verb and Wh subject cue– graphic and verbal (e.g., patient shown "eat" card while clinician says "eat," then shown "who" card while clinician says "who")	Produce appropriate subject after Wh subject cue (e.g., patient says "I")
	Wh object cue–graphic and verbal (e.g., patient shown "what" card while clinician says "what")	Produce appropriate object after Wh object cue (e.g., patient says "steak")

TABLE 7.2 Continued

LEVEL	STIMULI	RESPONSE
I	Verb and *Wh* cue–graphic and verbal (e.g., patient shown "eat" card while clinician says "eat," then shown "who" card while clinician says "who")	Respond with appropriate subject after *Wh* cue given (e.g., patients says "I")
		Generate S + V combination (e.g., patient says "I eat")
II-A	Verb–graphic and verbal (e.g., patient shown "eat" card while clinician says "eat")	Repeat verb (e.g., patient repeats "eat")
	Wh subject–graphic and verbal (e.g., patient shown "who" card while clinician says "who")	Repeat subject cue (e.g., patient repeats "who")
	Subject–graphic and verbal (e.g., patient shown "I" card while clinician says "I")	Repeat subject (e.g., patient repeats "I")
	Wh object cue–graphic and verbal (e.g., patient shown "what" card while clinician says "what")	Repeat *Wh* object cue (e.g., patient repeats "what")
	Object–graphic and verbal (e.g., patient shown "steak" card while clinician says "steak")	Repeat object (e.g., patient repeats "steak")
	S + V + O sentence– graphic and verbal (e.g., cards for "I eat steak" are shown to patient while clinician says "I eat steak")	Repeats S + V + O (e.g., patient repeats "I eat steak")

From Final Treatment Probe: (Same two pictures)
   Example 1: "That's a man . . . man's raking the leaves."
   Example 2: "Washing dishes . . . who . . . oh, yeah . . . that's a woman washing those dishes."

After about six months of work on the verbing program, Bob ceased to show positive changes in his communicative ability. Three consecutive probes indicated a leveling off of his performance at 5.2 words per utterance and a response latency of 4.3 seconds (see Figures 7.1, 7.2). He was extremely satisfied with his progress, however. He was also convinced that he had reaped every benefit from treatment and had reached maximum recovery. In helping to develop the final phase of treatment Bob had placed his priority on adequate verbal communication because he was communicating successfully, though minimally, with verbalizations. Gains made in the verbing program provided him with worthwhile strategies which actually worked in functional communication situations. Besides these gains he also improved his overall PICA score to the 84th percentile, an increase of 7 percentile points over the performance level prior to the verbing program (see Table 7.1).

SUMMARY

Maximum recovery? By what definition? How do we decide that a person will make no more progress or can no longer benefit from a structured treatment program? Termination from treatment is the end result of all client-clinician interactions, whether it is from choice or not. When termination is a matter of choice, it should be decided by the patient and the clinician together. The identification of the end-point of treatment was the concern of this case presentation. It seems that the most logical end-point of treatment is that point in time when the patient has benefited as much as possible from any therapeutic interaction. Maximum recovery, then, has occurred when significant improvement in communicative skills is no longer evident. The fallacy to this rule often rests in how we measure or determine "no further progress." Standardized testing provides only part of the answer. Communicative ability includes functional communication, complexity of content, length of messages, success of interactions, and many other elements.

Clinicians may need to become more sophisticated in delving into a patient's individual behavior to determine if there remains even one communicative behavior which could be changed substantially to promote a significant improvement in the ability to communicate. One simple strategy might assist a person's ability to communicate and should not be overlooked just for the sake of expediency. This case study provides one example of looking beyond the standardized tests for meaningful, measurable behavior that could be improved in order to assist functional communication.

REFERENCES

Loverso, F.L., Selinger, M., & Prescott, T.E. (1979). Applications of "verbing" strategies to aphasia treatment. In R.H. Brookshire (Ed.), *Clinical Aphasiology Conference Proceedings.* Minneapolis: BRK Publishers.

Davis, G.A. (1983). *A survey of adult aphasia.* Englewood Cliffs, NJ: Prentice-Hall.

Porch, B.E. (1967). *Porch Index of Communicative Ability.* Palo Alto, CA: Consulting Psychologists Press.

Porch, B.E., & Callahan, S. (1981). Making predictions about recovery. Is there HOAP? In R.H. Brookshire (Ed.), *Clinical Aphasiology Conference Proceedings.* Minneapolis: BRK Publishers.

Wertz, R.T., Deal, L., & Deal, J. (1980). Prognosis in aphasia: Investigation of the high-over (HOAP) and the short-direct (HOAP slope) method to predict change in PICA performance. In R.H. Brookshire (Ed.), *Clinical Aphasiology Conference Proceedings.* Minneapolis: BRK Publishers.

CHAPTER 8
Treatment of a Severely Aphasic Person
Michael Collins

> Collins describes the treatment course and outcome for a severely aphasic man. Early postonset the patient's neurologic residuals were so severe that he could not participate in formal treatment. When treatment did begin, the patient rejected all treatment tasks that did not promise speech. The author illustrates the importance of patience and appropriate timing of intervention efforts to achieve maximum results with severely aphasic persons, and the value of a total communication approach to overcome the severe verbal limitations of these patients.

1. What was the nature of the author's early assessment with the patient? What was learned through this series of observations? How did Collins deal with the patient's temper outbursts and reluctance to participate in treatment?
2. What was the primary goal in the early stage of treatment with the client? What was accomplished? Did this help prepare the patient for formal treatment? Why or why not?
3. What does the author mean by total communication? How did Collins employ a comprehension training program involving yes and no questions and make the patient think he was working on his speech? What are the benefits and problems in working on speech imitation drills while trying to conduct a total communication program?

INTRODUCTION

The patient described in this chapter is one of an unfortunately large number of people suffering from severe, chronic aphasia. Particularly during the first few months postonset the neurologic deficits of these individuals are so severe that their residual communication skills cannot be determined. As a consequence, they are frequently undertreated, mistreated, or not treated at all, and when they are ready to benefit from intensive speech and language treatment it may not be provided because the patient's insurance benefits have been exhausted.

Typically, in severe or global aphasia, both expression and reception are markedly involved and no single modality is strikingly better than another. In time, a characteristic profile of deficits may emerge that resembles a Broca's or Wernicke's aphasia. The profound deficits of these patients usually result from large lesions involving the distribution of the middle cerebral artery affecting frontal, temporal, and parietal lobes. Generally, more extensive lesions result in more severe and long-lasting deficits. Treatment of these deficits requires the patience and endurance of both clinician and patient, and the healing effects of time.

This case report describes the evolution of a severe aphasia, and the treatment for the aphasia, of a 56-year-old man. While our patient was globally aphasic initially, we witnessed the gradual emergence of a severe Broca's aphasia and some atypical responses to our treatment along the way.

THE CASE: MR. GREEN

The Patient

Mr. Green suffered a left hemisphere cerebrovascular accident and was taken to the hospital in serious condition. He remained in the intensive care unit for one week. Neurologic examination and brain-imaging procedures revealed a large infarct involving the left frontal and temporal lobes. Major neurologic residuals included a dense right hemianesthesia, a right homonymous hemianopsia, and a severe aphasia.

Initial Observation

Because of his early unstable medical and neurological status, Mr. Green was not seen until two weeks postonset. The first bedside evaluation provided little information. He was unresponsive and the responses that could elicited suggested that my presence was unwelcome. According to his family he was not angered easily or uncooperative before his stroke. I hoped that he would regain some semblance of his former good nature, but he tried my patience. He was not pressured to perform because it was felt that increased resistance would result. Instead, I quietly observed his communicative interactions with family and friends. Only occasionally was it possible to penetrate his barricade of anger and frustration with a question or instruction.

It was learned that Mr. Green was a proud, independent man who valued his privacy, independence, and family. I also learned that there was good reason for his anger and frustration. He was globally aphasic. His yes and no responses were inappropriate and inconsistent and except for a few automatic utterances he had no speech. His auditory comprehension was severely compromised.

Prognosis

Mr. Green's prognosis for substantial recovery of speech and language skills seemed bleak. This viewpoint was not shared immediately with him or his family, though it was clear that this information would become critical when Mr. Green went home to live with them. I discussed the nature of his aphasic deficits and stroke with them, shared bibliographic materials, and supported and encouraged their attempts to communicate with him. The family and his caregivers were provided with suggestions for communicating with him. I also tried to provide them with outlets for airing their frustration and fears.

Two weeks after his stroke, Mr. Green began active rehabilitation. His medical and neurological status had improved and so had his outlook. These changes permitted me to form a more complete picture of his deficits. However, his tolerance for me and his frustration level remained low. It was still necessary to continue to evaluate him informally through covert observation. At two weeks postonset, these tentative conclusions were reflected in my consult:

Patient referred for evaluation of speech and language deficits following a CVA November 16, 1980. Testing reveals the following:

Listening: Severely impaired. The patient is usually unable to follow instructions unless they are accompanied by gestures and/or appropriate pointing to objects or persons. With this supportive information he can follow some simple commands, but he cannot retain or follow commands involving more than one step. His auditory comprehension of single words appears to have improved since his stroke. He can point to single words presented auditorily 70% of the time. His comprehension is compounded by a severe premorbid binaural hearing loss. He was a reasonably good candidate for amplification but would not be able to participate in a hearing aid evaluation now. This evaluation will be deferred until the patient is able to respond adequately.

Reading: Severely impaired. The patient is able to recognize single words pronounced by the examiner at a level slightly above chance. He is unable to make associations among printed words and objects or pictures.

Writing: Writing is impossible to assess at this time because Mr. Green has rejected all attempts to test writing or copying ability. It is probable that writing is as impaired as speaking.

Speaking: Severely impaired. His speech consists of several recurring utterances such as "I never" and "Well I don't know." The phrases are automatic and are appropriate only by chance. His deficits in speech production are not due to weakness or paralysis despite a right lower facial weakness. He has a severe oral nonverbal apraxia and probably a severe apraxia of speech.

Impressions: Severe, global aphasia. He should improve in time but it is too early to tell how much improvement to expect. The extent and location of his lesion suggests that the evolution of his deficits will be from global aphasia toward what Mohr (1978) terms a "Big" Broca's aphasia, in which speech is telegraphic, halting, awkwardly articulated, and agrammatic. His prognosis is improved by his relative youth and premorbid intelligence. His severe hearing loss and coexisting medical problems are not in his favor, however. If he is to regain functional communication skills, treatment must be intense and protracted. This patient will be seen at least twice daily during the course of his hospitalization and make periodic reevaluations of his progress. Family counseling has begun to explain the nature of his language deficits and to ease any fears that, because his speech and language are impaired he has lost the ability to reason, and to guide them in their efforts to communicate with him.

Early Treatment

Mr. Green's psyche dictated that initial treatment sessions be brief. Few demands were placed on him to perform specific tasks. I began by assessing his ability to respond to questions and follow simple commands using whole body and axial movements. These included questions such as "Can you tell me the time?" and "What does the weather look like?" He was successful if these commands were presented in a conversational context, or if they involved body parts. For example, he could take his glasses off, open and close his eyes, and make a fist on command. Efforts to prompt him to attempt more structured treatment tasks, however, led to failure, frustration, and task rejection.

Despite conscientious efforts to avoid any type of formal evaluation or treatment of Mr. Green, by the second session I was barely able to coax him into the treatment room. By session five, no supplications had any effect, and he violently rejected assistance. I reluctantly agreed to terminate treatment until he was ready to participate. Three days later he voluntarily returned to the clinic, but on his terms. These terms included no formal testing and none of what he perceived as "treatment." Somehow I managed to establish a sort of rapport with him. He remained unwilling to work, but he did seem to enjoy coming to the clinic and interacting, provided I was very attentive and perceptive listener. Failure to communicate an idea was, to him, grounds for leaving. On one occasion he indicated this by writing "levc." In response, I wrote "leave?" and he responded "yes."

At six weeks postonset, this approach had yielded some dividends. Mr. Green was still globally aphasic, but the severity of his deficits had lessened. He could now repeat some real words. These consisted primarily of nouns and verbs. His auditory comprehension, reading, and writing had also improved. He could now follow some complex commands and identify, read, and copy a few single words. He also could play card games such as poker and "21."

Early Stage Treatment Summary

Reconnaissance and rapport-building efforts with Mr. Green were designed to obtain as much diagnostic and treatment planning information as possible without creating resistance to subsequent treatment and maladaptive behavioral sets. He was provided with nonthreatening tasks that he was willing to do and that allowed him some success. Efforts at this stage might be described as treatment by default, but this did not make them any less valuable. Moreover, Mr. Green's responses to us did not indicate that he should not have treatment, but that major rehabilitation efforts should wait until he was ready to participate in the process.

In early work with Mr. Green I wanted to make certain that both he and his wife understood the nature of his aphasia deficits and that treatment was available. It was clear that in the early postonset period he was not physically or emotionally ready for treatment or to make an informed choice. His past history indicated that if he decided to have formal treatment, he would work diligently. I was patient and perseverant; and I trusted that ultimately Mr. Green would make a decision about participating in treatment.

Mr. Green left the hospital, at his insistence, on January 4, when he was approximately seven weeks postonset. He, or his wife, was to call when he was ready for outpatient treatment. She called three weeks later. I agreed to see him twice weekly for a trial period of 60 days. When Mr. Green returned for his first outpatient visit, he was attentive and cooperative, and formal testing was begun that day.

Formal Treatment

The Porch Index of Communicative Ability (PICA) (Porch, 1967) was administered at four months postonset (see Figure 8.1). The test was ficult for Mr. Green and required nearly 70 minutes to administer. His Overall score was 8.66, which placed him at the 28th percentile. He obtained his highest subtest scores in the Gestural modality, but these only resulted in a 24th percentile ranking, the lowest of the three modalities. His highest modality percentile score was 32 for Verbals (raw score of 7.30), followed by 30 for Graphics (raw score of 6.55). From those modality and subtest scores, we attempted to predict future performance.

A conservative estimate, using Porch's HOAP slope formula (Porch, 1967), projected Mr. Green's performance to the 43rd percentile at six months postonset. These estimates are fairly reliable but his poor performance on the Verbal subtests except for repetition (5.0 on subtests I and IV, 6.2 on subtest IX) was of concern. Good performance on the repetition subtest, XII (13.00), and relatively good performance on Pantomime and Auditory Comprehension subtests alleviated concern somewhat, and his good copying ability gave additional reason for optimism.

A test for oral nonverbal and limb apraxia revealed significant deficits, although almost without exception performance improved with practice and instruction. Performance on the *Coloured Progressive Matrices* (Raven, 1956) was 24 correct of 36, which placed him between the 40th and 50th percentiles for normal men his age. The relationship between nonverbal problem-solving ability and language is controversial, but performance in chronic, global aphasia is usually much poorer, and I was more optimistic about his ability to learn and retain. Finally, the *Boston Diagnostic Aphasia Examination* (Goodglass & Kaplan, 1972) was administered. A subjective rating of the severity of his aphasia for the BDAE was one indicating "All communication is through fragmentary expression, and there is great need for inference, question, and guessing by the listener. The range of information that can be exchanged is limited, and the listener carries the burden of communication." His rating scale profile of speech characteristics was typical of that seen in Broca's aphasia.

Treatment Planning

Most approaches to aphasia treatment share common features and are guided by the same general principles. We are urged to begin treatment with simpler tasks on which the patient will be successful, and, either within the session or in some hierarchical fashion, move to more difficult tasks. Unfortunately, many of the easiest tasks for aphasic

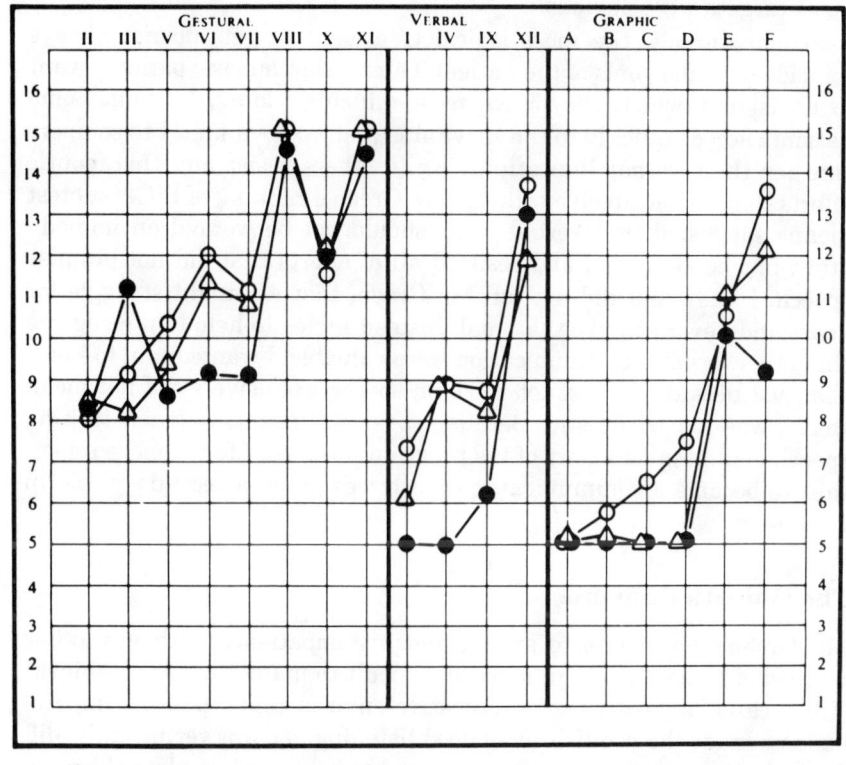

Figure 8.1 PICA subtest means for Gestural, Verbal, and Graphic modalities for Mr. Green at the beginning of treatment (2-28-81). Midway through treatment (10-15-81), and at the conclusion of formal treatment (2-25-82).

patients are not functional. Moreover, we have no good evidence that working on tasks such as matching, imitation, or copying allow for a hierarchical progression. Another principle of aphasia treatment stipulates that treatment should begin at a point on the patient's response curve where the patient just begins to experience difficulty. A ranking of subtest mean scores for a large sample of left-hemisphere damaged aphasic adults on the PICA (Porch, 1967) reveals that the easiest tasks on the PICA are matching object to object, matching picture to object, pointing to objects named, pointing to objects described by function, imitation, and copying. This ordering holds true for many but not all aphasic patients. Mr. Green's performance curve (see Figure 8.2), for example, was variable and atypical. When his PICA subtest means were ranked, however, a clear progression of difficulty emerged and treatment targets were obvious.

Unfortunately, the most logical treatment targets do not always coincide with the goals of the patient. Often, what aphasic patients want to do is that which they have most difficulty doing, talking. Some patients accede quickly to the inevitable and work valiantly to compensate for their verbal limitations, while others resist any therapeutic efforts that do not involve talking. Mr. Green's ranking of PICA subtest means suggested that verbal tasks should not be worked on immediately, but he struggled and resisted all of efforts that did not promise speech. I knew, but did not tell Mr. Green, that we might struggle for years and never achieve that goal. Instead I tried to help him recognize that other forms of communication were valuable. I wanted him to know that just because we did not work on speech exclusively did not mean that I was not optimistic. Because speaking meant so much to him, speech drill became a part of his program. Because I felt it more important to become a communicator, speech was given a secondary role in treatment.

The Patient's Response

Mr. Green's eagerness to speak, and his impatience with any other method of communication, made it difficult to maintain what Lubinski (1981) calls "a positive communicative environment," and his impetuousness made the acquisition of good listening and answering skills difficult. In these stages treatment was wrapped in a velvet glove. I began, tentatively at first, by trying to establish good listening skills, particularly for questions.

Initially, Mr. Green's yes and no responses were ambiguous and equivocal. He often said yes when he meant no or nodded his head yes and said no. When this occurred, it only increased his frustration. I tried to stabilize his yes and no responses. Because his auditory comprehension was better than verbal expression, and because reliable use of yes and no gave him a means of expressing understanding, agreement, or rejection, I began by having him point to cards labeled yes or no. Despite

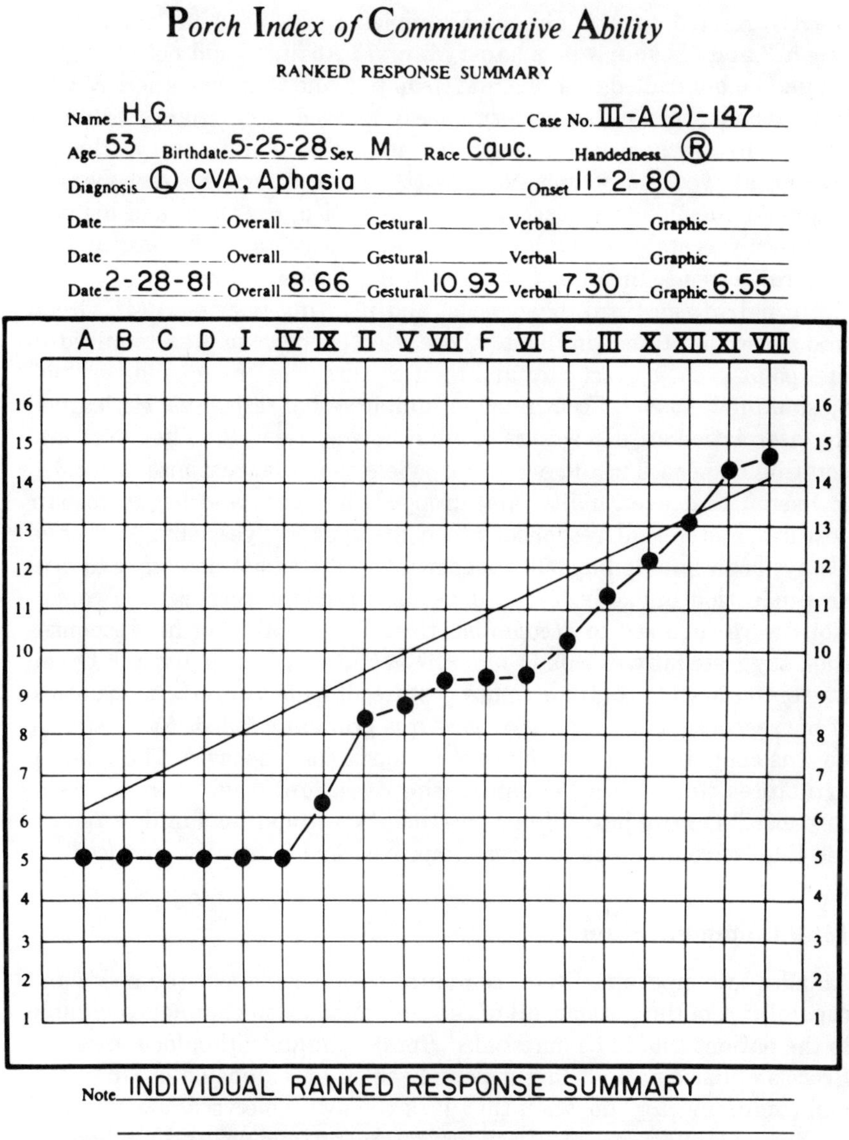

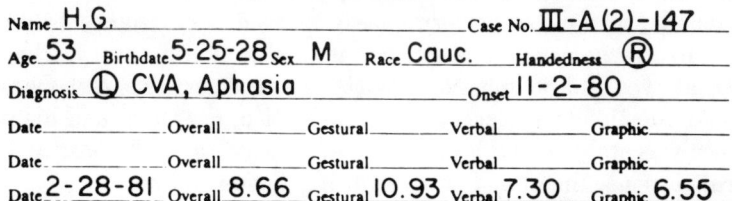

Figure 8.2 Individual ranked responses summary for Mr. Green after initial administration of the PICA on 2-28-81.

his resistance I insisted that pointing to either of these cards was the only response we would accept. He was also assured that this situation was only temporary. I acknowledged every response and corrected his mistakes, and I made sure that each stimulus and each response had a consequence. Questions were simple and direct and, whenever possible, directly related to Mr. Green. Examples were "Is your name Sam Green?" and "Is your wife's name Marge?" At first, I did not alternate yes and no but drilled first one, in sets of ten, and then the other. Within five sessions, his initial performance improved from chance to 90 to 100%. When responses had stabilized at this level of accuracy, I began to alternate yes and no questions. Within several sessions, responses to baselined questions were accurate 90 to 100% of the time, and his performance was stable enough to move to the next stage, the pairing of a gestural response (head nod) with pointing to yes and no.

In pairing gestural (head nods) and pointing responses Mr. Green was asked questions similar to those used earlier, but was required to first point to the correct card and then gesture "yes" by nodding or "no" by shaking his head. I continued to inhibit verbal responses. He learned the association in a few sessions but it was clear that gestural and pointing responses would eventually yield to verbal response. I decided to hasten that eventuality, and dropped the cards and began to pair gestural and verbal response. Since his spoken "yes" and "no" had always been intelligible, but undependable, it was not necessary to drill on production but only to stabilize his use of the responses. Two sessions were required to accomplish this. The stability of his responses then suggested it was safe to fade the gestural response, but Mr. Green was encouraged to continue to use gestures if he felt uncertain or unsure of his response. His reliance on gestures gradually faded. At all stages, he was cautioned against the use of imprudent responses. The guiding principles here were "consider the question" and "consider the response." On the basis of our treatment data and his family's report, the lines of communication were improved and frustration reduced.

Total Communication

An adequate program of total communication should suit the needs and capabilities of the patient; all of the communication channels available to the patient should be marshaled. Total communication for the severe Broca's aphasic patient might be viewed as an extension of what normal communicators do when they lack the available vocabulary to convey their ideas adequately. Drawing, gesturing, and writing can be used as adjuncts to spoken communication, and at times may be more powerful. In the beginning, it requires arduous, time-consuming instructions to get the patient to use a total communication system. Mr. Green was no exception.

Gesturing. In early sessions, I assessed spontaneous gestural ability informally in conversation, formally, in response to pictured or auditory stimuli, and imitatively. Intact gestures were incorporated into a corpus of gestures to be trained in therapy. Ten gesturable actions (e.g.. "eat," "drink," "smoke," and "listen") were selected for practice. When Mr. Green could not pantomime the desired response, real objects were used. When all gestures could be elicited on command, pantomime training began. Beginning with one gesture, I presented both spoken and gestured stimuli until that gesture could be produced reliably; then I expanded to two gestures, alternating between the two with fewer repetitions of each until he could alternate gestures successively through the final step. As he progressed, gestures were added and the process was repeated until all three gestures were firmly established.

Once Mr. Green had learned several gestures, he was encouraged to use them in response to questions. It was hoped that he would recognize the need for this and incorporate them into a program of total communication. Pointing became an integral part of his gestural training. Pointing, when used alone, conveys a message succinctly. When accompanied by verbal or nonverbal facilitators, such as facial expression, speech, or writing, it illuminates the message. Contextual pointing was incorporated in Mr. Green's total communication system by first establishing a clear, unequivocal gesture. Initially, the accuracy of the response was not nearly as important as the establishing of a clear response. He was asked to point to one object, or pictured object, with no foil. When the response was inadequate, he was requested to imitate the gesture until it was intact. As response adequacy increased, one foil was added and drilled on each step until adequacy was achieved. Next, the stimulus field was expanded by asking him to point to objects in the room, imitating my gestures when necessary. In the final stage, he was asked to look at a series of realistic, colored pictures, first pointing to objects I identified, and then pointing to corresponding items in the room. A similar procedure was used for conveying attributes such as color by having him point to objects of the same color as the target. The intent here was to teach him to use a point gesture to convey a simple message or an important attribute or to embellish an idea.

Drawing. When words or gestures fail, simple illustrations can be richly illustrative. Mr. Green retained the ability to draw simple pictures. He was encouraged to practice drawing at home and enlist his wife's help. He was asked to draw diagrams of his house, maps of his property and hometown, and frequently traveled routes. With his wife's assistance, he labeled these and brought them to the clinic, where we embellished, corrected, and drilled the labels, legends, and drawings, and tested his comprehension of them. He became skillful, and these abilities at one point became crucial. Nearly one year after his stroke, he was involved in an accident while driving to the clinic. Despite his limited speech, his drawing of the accident scene and sequence of events clearly conveyed his version of these events. That single event warranted continued emphasis on that mode of treatment.

Writing. Writing drill is a time-consuming activity for severely aphasic patients and is most efficient when much of the drill is done outside the clinic. Functional words that were salient to Mr. Green and the names of his family members were selected. Baseline performance rates were taken for three sessions. Then, two word lists were selected and equated for difficulty. A multiple baseline design was employed in which the treatment involved copying drill at home or a 20-word test followed by copying with assistance and corrections in the clinic. When a criterion of 80% correct was achieved for one list, we began treating the next list until all 40 words had been treated. Some generalization across lists occurred, but improvement for the untreated lists was never more than 30%, and at criterion level differences between treated and untreated stimuli were never less than 40%.

Speech. Mr. Green's relatively good repetition skill made it difficult to resist the temptation to work on speech production instead of other forms of communication. He was so eager to work on speech that homework became an important part of his treatment. Because his imitative ability was so good, we felt he was unlikely to practice his errors at home and he was given a Language Master. All words assigned for speech drill were written and recorded on cards. We encouraged him to practice as much as he could, and asked him to keep a daily log of practice time.

Auditory Comprehension

Auditory comprehension seems to improve with or without treatment, although specific treatment enhances it. I suspect, although I cannot demonstrate it, that the carefully controlled auditory stimulation within the yes-no programming, in which Mr. Green was required to consider the stimulus carefully and respond to each stimulus numerous times, was beneficial. Because auditory comprehension was initially his best modality and seemed to be improving without direct intervention, we chose not to treat it extensively.

Combining Modalities for Total Communication

Once Mr. Green had established some facility in gesturing, drawing, writing, and spelling, "PACE" therapy (Davis & Wilcox, 1981), a program designed to allow the communication of new information in any available modality, was introduced. To facilitate this process, Mr. Green was provided with a pencil and paper, and these tools were treated as natural extensions of the communication process. Using realistic, colored cards that depicted only one clear action, he was asked to describe the action in any or all of the modalities open to him. Responses that communicated the action were accepted. These responses were not necessarily "accurate" linguistically but were communicative. When the response communicated his thoughts, he was reinforced by modeling of his response and letting him know he was successful. When he failed to communicate, an acceptable response was modeled for him to imitate. As his competence improved, the vocabulary was expanded, and when he could communicate approximately ten actions, I began to focus exchanges on more natural communicative topics. The clinician and patient alternated serving as speaker and listener. As his ability improved we began to exchange information about his activities and interests, and involved his family, particularly his wife, in the treatment. Themes that evolved included his family, hobbies, travel, and current events. In our clinic sessions, he was asked to identify one or two themes for discussion, or we selected a theme. As the theme was developed, central and related descriptors were incorporated.

In these early PACE sessions, much of the burden of communication was on the clinician, but in subsequent sessions I transferred as much of that burden to him as he would accept. He accepted the challenge.

Results

Mr. Green's treatment became sporadic after the first year. With his increased physical recovery and added leisure time, he resumed many of his previous activities, including travel, and frequently could not find the time for treatment. We obliged his intermittent treatment schedule and assessed his progress with intermittent testing. It was clear that he had improved; Family, staff, and those in our clinic noted it. Unfortunately, we were unable to capture much of the improvement with formal testing, although the testimony from our probes of treated and untreated stimuli is available. Performance on formal tests, specifically the PICA, is shown in Figure 8.1. Mr. Green never reached the predicted level of the 43rd percentile, but he came close. Because he is a tenacious worker, he appears to do better than that. But I suspect that no formal measure could capture this tenaciousness or depict his achievements.

Follow-up

At five years postonset Mr. Green is still making progress. He frequently delights us with a new word, sometimes including a very descriptive Anglo-Saxon verb to describe the wonders to be seen on late night television programming via satellite dish. He recently discovered our microcomputer and comes to clinic more frequently. He is presently making slow progress on a program to improve spelling and reading comprehension. It is hoped that Mr. Green will continue to improve as time progresses. He seems to know, perhaps better than his clinicians, his communicative needs, but he sometimes relies on us to help him achieve them. By responding to his needs and by documenting the effects of our response, we advance his cause and that of our profession.

REFERENCES

Davis, A.G., & Wilcox M.J. (1981). Incorporating parameters of natural conversation in aphasia treatment. In R. Chapey (Ed.), *Language intervention strategies in adult aphasia*. Baltimore: Williams & Wilkins.

Goodglass, H., & Kaplan, E. (1972). *The assessment of aphasia and related disorders*. Philadelphia: Lea and Febiger.

Lubinski, R. (1981). Environmental language intervention. In R. Chapey (Ed.), *Language intervention strategies in adult aphasia*. Baltimore: Williams & Wilkins.

Mohr, J. (1978). Broca aphasia: Pathologic and clinical. *Neurology, 28,* 311–324.

Porch, B. (1967). *The Porch Index of Communication Ability*. Palo Alto, CA: Consulting Psychologists Press.

Raven, J. (1956). *Coloured Progressive Matrices*. London: H.K. Lewis.

CHAPTER 9
Aphasia and Severe Apraxia of Speech: Charting the Treatment Course

James L. Aten

> *Aphasic patients often persist in their quest to reestablish verbal communication when this feat may not be attainable. Aten describes the treatment of a client whose aphasia was compounded by a severe oral and verbal apraxia. The author illustrates the importance of systematically treating and measuring client performance on tasks designed to facilitate verbal production. He offers clinical insights as to why some brain-injured individuals may not be candidates for verbal communication approaches.*
>
> 1. What clinical evidence does Aten provide that suggests that the client's apraxic deficits are unlikely to change as a consequence of treatment?
> 2. Describe how the client's aphasic (language) deficits resolve in the course of treatment. How does this compare with what occurs with his verbal production problems?
> 3. What disparities are noted in the client's speaking performance in demanding and more relaxed communicative situations? Why? How would the severity of the patient's verbal deficits differ in both contexts? How might this be used to plan treatment for a severely apraxic client?
> 4. Would Aten's client have become a functional communicator if a nonverbal treatment approach were used? Why or why not?

Introduction

Many aphasia clinicians have treated patients similar to the case presented in this chapter. These individuals suffer left-hemisphere cerebrovascular accidents (CVA) with resulting right hemiparesis, aphasia, and severe apraxia of speech. Typically, they show some early spontaneous recovery of auditory comprehension, single word reading and writing, but despite an intense desire to talk again, fail to regain functional speaking ability. Clinicians often describe these patients as having "moderate aphasia with good reception complicated by severe oral apraxia and apraxia of speech." The case presented in this chapter was such a patient.

Clients who present both severe language and verbal production deficits pose a serious dilemma for the clinician. This dilemma involves making a decision as to what to treat first—the language deficit, the verbal communication deficit, both deficits, or in some instances, to abandon attempts to improve verbal communication entirely and utilize an alternative output channel. The situation is further compounded if the patient insists that "he learn to talk" again, and, through pressure from family, friends, and others, that treatment will not be successful unless he talks.

It is hoped that the chronicle of this case's treatment will assist clinicians in selecting the most efficacious treatment path. If practicing, and soon to be practicing, clinicians are able to chart treatment directions quickly and to identify the problems that prevent communication from occurring by reading this chapter, the time spent in documenting the treatment of this case will be well justified.

BACKGROUND INFORMATION

John, age 52, was traveling to the East Coast when he suffered a sudden onset of aphasia and right hemiplegia on October 8, 1982. A medical examination confirmed that he had suffered a left thromboembolic CVA. He had retired from jobs as an automobile salesman and truck driver in 1980 because of health problems secondary to diabetes and hypertension. John had also manifested some prestroke depression following a divorce and from the pressures of trying to raise two teenage girls by himself. The only other medically significant event occurred some twenty years earlier. This event involved a car accident that resulted in a brief period of unconsciousness and loss of his right eye. No permanent neurological residuals secondary to the accident could be found, but the possibility of earlier right frontal damage was a consideration, despite the fact that CT scans after his stroke revealed only left temporal-parietal damage and disruption of blood flow from the left middle cerebral artery.

Immediately following his CVA, John received some limited speech and physical therapy at the Dallas VA Medical Center. He regained the ability to walk with the aid of a cane but did not recover function of his right arm. His Overall mean score on the *Porch Index of Communicative Ability* (PICA) (Porch, 1967) at one month post-CVA placed him at the 35th percentile in comparison to a large random sample of left-hemisphere damaged adults. His performance on the auditory subtests of the PICA was essentially intact, but he had some problems understanding the prepositional directions of the reading subtests (e.g., "Put this card on the one used for fixing hair"). His mean score on the PICA Graphic tests put him at the 52nd percentile, but his performance on Verbal subtests of the PICA was markedly impaired (1st percentile). Subsequently, John was released, returned home to California, and requested speech and language treatment as an outpatient at the Long Beach VA Medical Center. In January of 1983, John agreed to become a subject in a Veterans Administration Cooperative Study (Wertz et al., 1984) of treatment of aphasia. He was administered an extensive battery of tests when he entered the study (intake) and at six-week intervals for the next six months (see Tables 9.1, 9.2, 9.3). This battery included the PICA; *Boston Diagnostic Aphasic Exam* (BDAE) (Goodglass & Kaplan, 1972); *Reading Comprehension Battery for Aphasia* (RCBA) (LaPointe & Horner, 1979); *Communication Abilities in Daily Living* (CADL) (Holland, 1980); *Token Test* (Spreen & Benton, 1969); and the *Coloured Progressive Matrices* (RCPM) (Raven, 1962). He was assigned randomly to the deferred treatment group (12 weeks) and began receiving eight hours of individual traditional speech and language treatment in April 1983. John's test scores for the intake six-week and twelve-week evaluations improved minimally without treatment, probably reflecting continuing spontaneous recovery.

THE CASE: JOHN

Traditional Treatment

From April 24, 1983 until July 15, 1983, John was provided 8 hours of speech and language treatment each week. This focused on ameliorating deficits in all language modalities.

Auditory Comprehension. Although John had relatively good auditory comprehension ability, his severe limitations in verbal production made it impossible for him to respond other than by means of a written or a pointing response. Comprehension tasks used in treatment involved pictures, printed words, and objects. In the initial phases of treatment, comprehension training stressed left-right discrimination (e.g., "Touch your right shoulder"), prepositional relationships (e.g., "Put the pencil on top of the card"), temporal sequencing (e.g., "I'll say three words: Houston, Miami, and Cleveland. Show me on the map the three cities I named"), and answering yes and no questions about the paragraphs read to him. These activities began with simple straightforward questions and progressed accordingly in terms of length and complexity. Another task that was useful to John was to read a story to him describing a series of functional relationships (e.g., man getting in a car, driving to the store, making a purchase, etc.) and then asking him to arrange the story sequence using objects or pictures. By the end of his period of traditional treatment, John had functional comprehension and could understand five to seven word sentences with 80% accuracy.

Reading. Treatment of John's reading deficits was carried out at the sentence and paragraph levels. This involved having John read sentences and/or paragraphs and respond with yes or no answers or choose from a multiple choice format about what he had read. While he read slowly and had difficulty retaining lengthy passages, he usually performed accurately, and was able to grasp the functional significance of what he had read.

Writing. Treatment of John's writing difficulties focused on improving spelling and single words. Practice words were selected that would help him compensate for his severe verbal deficits by allowing him to express everyday needs graphically. Particularly useful were frequently used items such as coffee, eggs, and money concepts (e.g., price, cost, dollar, check). Some effort was made to expand his written single word productions into longer phrases and sentences. Occasionally this procedure resulted in a two to three word phrase in response to an action picture (e.g., man eat food) or the writing of longer directions presented auditorily. The greatest benefit of writing of longer directions was that John learned to write single words to express many of his daily living needs.

Verbal Production. John had almost no ability to produce speech. Treatment of his verbal production deficits began with simple imitation drills intended to elicit simple CV syllables. Because he was markedly impaired in the fine motor control of his tongue, lips, and jaw, only targets requiring the grossest of articulatory movements were practiced. Typically the consonants /m/, /p/, /b/, and /w/ were combined with a vowel, so as to form a simple word (e.g., my, pie, bye, we, woe). Selection of items for imitation drill was predicated on John's success in practice and included those items that could be successfully cued with printed words, or "cloze" techniques (e.g., I want a piece of apple _____)." Intensive clinician modeling and instruction were provided. In addition, John was encouraged to try to reduce his abrupt voice onset and to initiate production in a more relaxed manner.

After 12 weeks of traditional treatment, only portions of which were spent in improving verbal production, John could produce simple consonant-vowel syllables on imitation tasks (80–95% success), in response to questions (80–85% success), and when reading single words (60–75% success). These syllables usually contained a bilabial consonant (/p/, /b/, /m/, /w/) and a vowel. Productions were accurate, but he often substituted the voiced consonants /b/ and /m/ for /p/.

Results of Traditional Treatment

In 12 weeks of traditional aphasia treatment John made small gains in some areas and showed no improvement in others. Table 9.1 shows his test scores for the PICA, BDAE, RCBA, CADL, *Token Test* and RCPM at the time of his intake evaluation and at successive six-week intervals. During the first 12 weeks John received no treatment but was simply brought in for testing every six weeks. This was a condition he agreed to in order to enter the study.

Performance Stability. John's overall percentile ranking (47th percentile) on the PICA at the time of his intake evaluation reflects a significant gain from his earliest testing (35th percentile) at the Dallas VA Medical Center. This result suggests that considerable spontaneous recovery took place between his leaving Texas and arriving in Long Beach. Comparison of test scores for the intake evaluation and the 6 week and 12 week evaluation points (see Table 9.1) indicate that John's performance stabilized over the time when he did not receive treatment. For example, his PICA overall score put him at the 47th percentile at intake, the 52nd after six weeks, and the 51st after 12 weeks. Similar trends are shown on the other measures of the assessment battery during the deferred treatment period.

Lack of Treatment Effects. John's stable test scores over the 12 week period in which he received no treatment provide a baseline against which to measure the effects of his 12 weeks of traditional treatment. Table 9.1 clearly reveals that the effects of this treatment were negligible and results are disappointing for even the most optimistic of clinicians. John's scores on the PICA dropped, as did those for the RCBA, *Token Test*, and RCPM. Scores for the CADL increased slightly as did those on the BDAE (this occurred after a drop in performance from 12 to 18 weeks). Tables 9.2 and 9.3 provide a more definitive analysis of changes within modalities for the PICA and BDAE,

TABLE 9.1
Test Battery Scores for 12-Week Period of No Treatment Followed by 12 Weeks of Intensive Treatment (Cooperative Aphasia Study #110)

			MEASURE			
TEST DATES (Highest possible)	PICA PERCENTILES OVERALL (99%)	BOSTON DIAGNOSTIC APHASIA EXAMINATION (556)	READING COMPREHENSION BATTERY FOR APHASIA (100)	CADL (136)	TOKEN TEST (163)	RAVENS (36)
Intake	47	216	75	104	144	27
6 weeks	52	235	87	95	153	29
12 weeks*	51	239	88	101	152	33
18 weeks	51	217	74	111	145	35
24 weeks	48	243	76	114	145	28

*Treatment initiated

TABLE 9.2
PICA Scores from Intake Through the 24th Week Evaluation by Modalities

TEST DATES	OVERALL	AUDITORY (15 possible)	READING	GRAPHIC	VERBAL
Intake	47%	14.7	12.9	72%	20%
6 weeks	52%	14.8	13.8	82%	21%
12 weeks	51%	15.0	14.6	78%	18%
18 weeks	51%	14.9	14.0	75%	21%
24 weeks	48%	14.2	13.3	73%	21%

TABLE 9.3
BDAE Scores from Intake Through the 24th Week Evaluation by Modalities

TEST DATES (Highest possible)	OVERALL (556)	AUDITORY (119)	READING (46)	WRITING (101)	ORAL (290)
Intake	216	111	37	66	2
6 weeks	235	114	37	78	6
12 weeks*	239	116	37	74	12
18 weeks	217	111	35	59	12
24 weeks	243	114	36	73	20

*Treatment initiated

but these data also support the prior observations of stable performance before treatment initiation and negligible treatment effects.

Communicative Status. Fortunately, John showed some benefits of treatment that were not reflected in his formal test scores. His auditory comprehension and reading had improved to functional levels. He communicated more of his needs by writing single words, but this feat necessitated much probing and cueing by the listener and was a time-consuming process. John was, however, persistent in his efforts to communicate his thoughts. He wrote single words and supplemented these with crude gestures, "grunts," and facial expressions. He remained, however, a verbal cripple, limited to the use of a few single-syllable words such as "my," "bye," "I," "love," and "pie." Additional testing in the clinic showed John's motor speech impairments to be even more basic. He was essentially unable to produce a stream of air without phonating. When asked to sigh, whistle, or to blow out a match, he tended to "grunt" or let air escape through his nose. He could not purse or retract his lips consistently nor could he bite his lower lip precisely. It was difficult for him to elevate his tongue without looking in a mirror and/or assisting its elevation with his finger. Raising the back of the tongue (as required in production of /k/ or /g/) was impossible. Many movements that could not be elicited voluntarily were observed during automatic acts such as swallowing, eating, and brushing his teeth. To summarize, John demonstrated severe oral apraxia in addition to his apraxia of speech and no significant dysarthria. His gestural system was simplistic, incomplete, and not functional. He communicated largely by writing single words requiring the listener to play twenty questions to elicit information on current or past events, feelings, and so forth.

REFOCUSING TREATMENT

It was readily apparent from the limited results of treatment designed to improve John's verbal production that he would need to produce more than voiced bilabials to be a functional speaker. A decision was made to put more emphasis on ameliorating his oral apraxia and his apraxia of speech but to focus this treatment on more basic aspects of speech production.

Self-Assisted Treatment

A videotape was made using a selected list of John's key words. On the tape a clinician presented a printed word and said the word three times. Visual cues for phonetic placement were provided by using the zoom lens of the camera to focus directly on the clinician's face as the word was being said. John came to the clinic and practiced by himself using the videotape as a model. Clinician-administered checks were taken weekly to assess his progress in producing the list of key words and to determine the generalization of his videotaped assisted practice on a list of nonpracticed words. John was able to produce 80% to 90% of the words on the practiced list successfully without the facilitating cues provided by videotape, but there was little evidence of generalization of this practice to untreated words.

Other Efforts

In an attempt to break up John's severely apraxic struggles and to increase his phonemic repertoire, two other procedures were attempted.

MIT. John was given a trial of *Melodic Intonation Therapy* (Sparks & Holland, 1976) to determine whether this treatment might reduce struggle and facilitate more prosodic, fluent, and hopefully intelligible productions. MIT was not successful. John was unable to produce intoned sequences. His efforts consisted of two or three abrupt vocalizations which were highly perseverative, characterized by struggle, and had minimal tonal variation.

Automatic Speech. Many apraxic patients can produce automatic sequences (e.g., counting, alphabet, days of week) without "thinking about what they are doing" but cannot produce single elements of automatic sequences voluntarily. Although John had considerable difficulty with automatic speech tasks in formal testing, his performance on these tasks was somewhat better (longer, relaxed, more intelligible utterances) in an informal clinical setting. An attempt was made to capitalize on the disparity between the formal test situation and clinical performance to see if a breakthrough might occur by improving production of automatic speech.

When attempting to produce an automatic sequence (e.g., counting to 10). John was instructed to delay responding until he was relaxed and ready. He was encouraged to practice lip, tongue, and jaw exercises at home in front of a mirror and to try to extend the range of each movement (e.g., tongue protrusion) as much as possible. In the clinic these exercises were combined with breath flow. For example, the movement of biting the lower lip in combination with breath flow assisted John in producing the word "five." Eventually he was able to count to 10 and to say the days of the week with 75% intelligibility, but he continued to substitute voiced for voiceless consonants (e.g., "bour" for "four") even when specifically reminded not to do so. Encouragement to speak in a more relaxed fashion resulted in softer vocalizations that were emitted with less effort and struggle on automatic speech tasks. However, if John practiced excessively or if his attention was specifically directed to the task, his speech became labored and phonemic accuracy deteriorated. Without constant reminders and modeling John was unable to use this relaxed style of production outside the clinic. It was therefore decided to direct treatment toward an even more basic process, that of establishing respiratory control for production of voiceless continuants.

Continuancy Training

The objective of this treatment program was to develop John's ability to shape a voiceless air stream in order to produce the fricative continuant consonants /f/, /s/, /θ/, and /ç/ in CV and CVC words. Preliminary steps in working towards this objective involved (1) having John produce the glottal consonant /h/ in combination with a vowel (e.g., he, ha, ho, hoo) in a whispered syllable and (2) directing the voiceless air stream orally. The latter involved activities such as blowing out matches and blowing whistles and then having John constrict the air stream using tongue and lip movements so as to achieve frication type sounds.

To assess the patient's ability to produce the fricative consonants /f/, /θ/, /s/, and /ʃ/ a single subject design similar to that recently reported by LaPointe (1984) was employed. Forty CV and CVC words were selected, 10 each beginning with each of the four consonants. Twenty words were assigned to a treatment list; 20 were assigned to a no treatment list. Words were selected to provide nearly equal occurrence of vowels and final consonants, and the treated and nontreated lists were counterbalanced. These precautions were taken to rule out the influence of phonetic context on production accuracy for the four initial target phonemes.

Baseline measures of production accuracy for the target phenomes were obtained. John produced no phoneme accurately during baseline except the /f/ which was produced infrequently. In treatment John was provided intensive multimodal stimulation in the form of a printed word, visual modeling ("Watch me"), and auditory stimulation. Models were eliminated when John could respond to the printed word cue alone. Throughout treatment he was provided with substantial verbal instruction and clinician feedback.

In the first phase of his treatment encompassing 14 sessions, 50% of the time was allocated to working on /f/; 25% to /θ/; 12% to /ʃ/ and 0% to /s/. Production accuracy was recorded by the clinician as follows: /f/ = 70%; /θ/ = 65%; /ʃ/ = 60%; /s/ = 0%. It should be emphasized that these levels of accuracy were attained with intensive stimulation, clinician modeling, and feedback.

In a second phase of continuancy training the amount of time allocated to working on the four phonemes was reversed (/s/ = 50%; /ʃ/ = 25%; /θ/ = 12%; /f/ = 0%). Treatment procedures were identical including the number (14) of treatment sessions.

To assess the transfer of treatment to a nontreatment situation, and to determine the generalization of practice on the treated list to the nontreated list of words, perceptual judgments of tape-recorded verbal productions were made by graduate students in speech pathology. John produced the forty words from each list when presented with printed word cues. The judges were unaware of the treatment design and target words. They were instructed to listen to the word and circle one cf the four target phonemes which were produced in the initial position of each word. They were permitted to circle a question mark choice when they could not determine which phoneme they had heard in a particular word.

Results. After phase one of continuancy treatment /f/ was the only phoneme perceived by the graduate student judges beyond a chance level (26%). Similar results occurred after the second treatment phase; /f/ was the only phoneme perceived (32%). In both judging sessions all other phonemes were identified at less than chance levels, or judges were unable to discriminate the phoneme produced. Results indicated that direct intensive treatment had failed to improve John's production accuracy on the four voiceless continuants with the exception of /f/ and this occurred at slightly more than a chance level.

WHAT CAN WE LEARN FROM JOHN?

As stated eariler, John represents a type of patient frequently encountered by clinicians. Typically, such patients are anxious to talk again. Clinicians are equally eager to get them talking again and many work very hard to accomplish this. Unfortunately, we do not always succeed as John so vividly demonstrates. This patient has much to teach us, however, about the expectations we have of our clients and treatment techniques.

Verbal Communication. Not all patients should be expected to regain functional verbal communication. Individuals who are several months postonset who cannot produce some automatic speech may have a poor overall prognosis for regaining functional speech. While the presence of automatic speech does not necessarily indicate a favorable prognosis, it does provide a "starting point" to attack the problems of severe apraxia. John had no automatic speech. Attempts to establish automatic sequential productions failed. Efforts to establish rudimentary verbal skills at even more basic levels fared similarly. Apraxia, when severe and affecting both nonverbal and speech movement patterns, is not always amenable to treatment. The complex coordinations of synchronizing air flow and voicing with tongue-lip movements were simply not acquired despite intensive practice.

Performance Disparities. John performed much differently in relaxed, informal, contextually-rich, reinforcing situations, including real-life settings, than he did on formal test measures, direct treatment exercises, and the various clinical investigative measures designed to assess his response to treatment. All speaking tasks of a confrontative nature negatively affected his speaking performance, but in less pressured situations he produced some surprises. For example, in group therapy when asked where he had lived, he stated "Washington, D.C."

When he was encouraged to answer questions about himself using the relaxed speaking style recommended when working on automatic sequence production, he gave intelligible replies to stimuli such as "How old are you?" and "Who is going to win the election?" His self-reports indicated that he ordered "ham 'n eggs" in the canteen and received the food requested. At the post office he was successful in saying "I want money order." Finally, while John showed little improvement on most of the language tests, he did improve markedly on his CADL performance. His CADL score (see Table 9.1) was 114 when he ended traditional treatment in the VA cooperative study. His most recent performance was 124. Since the CADL is a less confrontative test than the PICA, BDAE, or RCBA, it may be a better measure of treatment efficacy with patients such as John. A previous study by Aten, Caligiuri and Holland (1982) found the CADL to be more sensitive to change than the PICA in chronic aphasic patients receiving functionally oriented treatment. Perhaps because the CADL gives the patient credit for successful communication via any modality or modality combination and partial credit for responses that are "in the ballpark," it should be the measure of choice for individuals such as John. We can conclude, however, that confrontative communicative situations tended to compound John's problems and did not reflect a true picture of how he communicated in the real world.

Measurement of Treatment Effects. A single subject design study was conducted to measure the effects of our treatment with John. Unfortunately, the outcome of the investigation of his ability to establish voiceless continuancy told us that we were "beating a dead horse" with respect to reestablishing verbal skills. Knowing the answer to an important question, however, is better than giving the patient prolonged periods of speech exercise and drill based on "hope." Although our study did not yield positive results, it did help us chart a course oriented toward enhancing John's communication rather than improving his speech.

Future Directions

With patients like John we may need to examine the use of alternative communication modes early in treatment, while accepting and reinforcing the speech these persons do produce in nonconfrontative situations. It is unlikely, however, that John would have accepted this early in treatment. He attended treatment religiously because he "wanted to speak," and early attempts to encourage the use of gestures were not successful. Time, and a growing awareness by John and clinicians who will perhaps give it "another go," will provide the answer as to whether he will accept being a nonverbal communicator or continue to be frustrated.

ACKNOWLEDGMENT

Appreciation is expressed to the Veterans Administration Cooperative Studies Programs and to Dr. R. T. Wertz, Principal Investigator, Cooperative Study Project #110 for funding that supported a portion of the testing and treatment reported in this chapter. I wish also to express thanks to Amy Clark and to Yvonne Fortine who carefully administered the treatment during various periods of the project. Thanks also to the Long Beach VA Medical Center for its overall support of the treatment program.

REFERENCES

Aten, J., Caligiuri. M., & Holland, A. (1982). The efficacy of functional communication therapy for chronic aphasic patients. *Journal of Speech and Hearing Disorders, 47.* 93-96.

Goodglass, H., & Kaplan, E. (1972). *The assessment of aphasia and related disorders.* Philadelphia: Lea and Febiger.

Holland. A.L. (1980). *Communicative Abilities in Daily Living.* Austin. TX: PRO-ED.

LaPointe, L. (1984). Sequential treatment of split lists. In J. Rosenbek, M. McNeil, & A.F. Aronson (Eds.), *Apraxia of speech.* San Diego: College-Hill Press.

LaPointe, L., & Horner, J. (1979). *Reading Comprehension Battery for Aphasia.* Tigard, OR: C.C. Publications.

Porch, B. E. (1967). *Porch Index of Communicative Ability.* Palo Alto, CA: Consulting Psychologists Press.

Raven, J.C. (1962). *Coloured Progressive Matrices.* London: H.K. Lewis.

Sparks, R., & Holland, A.L. (1976). Method: Melodic intonation therapy for aphasia. *Journal of Speech and Hearing Disorders, 41,* 287-297.

Spreen, O., & Benton, A.L. (1969). *Neuro Sensory Center Comprehensive Examination for Aphasia.* Victoria, BC: University of Victoria, Neuropsychology Laboratory.

Wertz, R.T., LaPointe, L., Weiss, D., Holland, A., Brookshire, R., Aten, J., Kurtzke, J., Garcia, L., & members of the VA Cooperative Study #110 Group, (1984). *A comparison of clinic, home, and deferred treatment programs for aphasia.* Unpublished study.

CHAPTER 10

Evolution of Communication in a Traumatically Head Injured Patient with Aphasia

Reg L. Warren

>Warren describes the nine year recovery of a 34-year-old man following a traumatic head injury. The client remained speechless for nearly four and one-half years. During this time, treatment emphasized a total communication approach and the client relied heavily on use of the Handi-Voice 110, an augmentative device. Then the client's speech suddenly returned. Treatment continued emphasizing combined use of speech and the augmentative system. The unusual recovery course of this case provides an opportunity to make some inferences about augmentative communication systems and their impact on speech and language.
>
>1. How does Warren describe the client's aphasia? What evidence does he provide to support his diagnostic impressions?
>2. Describe the major aspects of the client's total communicative program. What were some of the reasons the author decided to try an augmentative system with him? Describe the training with the Handi-Voice.
>3. What were the facilitating effects of Handi-Voice instruction on the client's written and verbal communication? How does Warren explain the client's sudden return to speech? Summarize the author's comments with regard to the use of augmentative devices with the brain injured.

BACKGROUND OF THE PATIENT

Jim was a bright, articulate PhD student in the biological sciences. He had published some research and was considered one of the top students in his program by his professors. On September 22, 1975, he was hit by an automobile while riding a bicycle. He suffered a severe closed head injury and immediate respiratory arrest. An emergency tracheotomy was performed and a burrhole was subsequently placed in his skull to decrease intercranial pressure. Neuroradiographic studies revealed that Jim had incurred subdural and intracerebral hematomas in the left parietal area. It was suspected that there had been some bruising of the right hemisphere as well, and that bleeding had occurred in both right and left cerebral hemispheres. Two weeks later Jim underwent a left parietal craniotomy. He was in a coma for eight weeks. When he regained consciousness, he exhibited a dense right hemiplegia, diplopia, and total loss of communication skills. In November of 1975 (two months postonset), Jim was transferred to the St. Louis, Missouri Veterans Administration Medical Center. The admitting physician's note described him as follows: "The patient does not speak or groan. He does not follow commands but looks about the room in all directions. He defends himself by moving his left arm in response to painful stimuli."

THE CASE: JIM

Initial Evaluation

Jim was seen for evaluation by speech-language pathology at approximately four months postonset. The *Porch Index of Communicative Ability* (PICA) (Porch, 1971), was administered as a part of a comprehensive evaluation. Jim's Overall mean score on the PICA was 7.15 which placed him at the 31st percentile in a large random sample of bilaterally damaged patients. He presented severe communicative deficits in all language modalities but his most noticeable impairment was a total absence of speech (see Table 10.1).

When Jim tried to speak, he opened his mouth and waved his left hand aimlessly. He did not phonate and no articulatory movements were observed. He was cooperative, attentive, and tried to perform all tasks requested by the examiner. He used facial expressions and crude gestures to show the examiner when he was confused, needed a stimulus repetition, or was frustrated by task demands. Jim was diagnosed as having severe head trauma syndrome, with a focal aphasia and severe oral and verbal apraxia. His performance in auditory, reading, and writing tasks suggested that if he could speak, his aphasia type would be Broca's.

TABLE 10.1
Test Number, Months Postonset (MPO), Date, Overall and Modality Scores Based on Bilateral Percentile Equivalents

NO.	MPO	DATE	OVERALL	%	GESTURAL	%	VERBAL	%	GRAPHIC	%
1	4.0	1/14/76	7.15	31	10.47	45	2.0	2	6.15	56
2	9.0	6/21/76	9.30	55	13.86	89	2.0	2	8.10	75
3	35.0	8/23/78	10.21	63	13.97	90	4.75	20	8.83	78
4	52.0	1/07/80	10.82	69	13.86	88	9.48	48	7.67	74
5	55.5	4/23/80	11.25	73	13.59	82	11.73	62	7.82	86
6	60.0	9/04/80	12.72	87	13.93	90	13.15	76	10.83	76
7	107.0	8/10/84	11.85	75	13.43	78	12.45	67	8.20	56

TREATMENT

Total Communication

From 4 to 9 months postonset Jim was seen for 122 speech and language therapy sessions. Treatment stressed total communication and focused on three areas: (a) developing a gestural communication system, (b) stimulating phonation and articulatory movements, and (c) improving functioning in reading, writing, and listening.

Gesturing. Amer-Ind Gestural Code is a hand code derived from a manual signing system of the American Indian. The system contains several hundred concrete, easily acquired, highly interpretable signs that have been found to be useful with persons who are incapable of verbal communication (Skelly, 1979).

Jim was given practice on a set of 70 gestures from the Amer-Ind Program. After 66 sessions of individual instruction, observers familiar with the signing system could recognize his gestures approximately 80% of the time. Those who were unfamiliar with the system, however, had difficulty interpreting his signs primarily because of the inconsistency of his limb movements and his impaired sequential organization of the gestural movements. Moreover, Jim did not use these gestures spontaneously in communicative interactions outside of the clinic. When he did attempt to communicate with gestures, he tended to embellish his movements with unrelated movements that confused observers.

Phonation and Articulation. To stimulate voluntary phonation Jim was directed to place his fingers on the clinician's larynx while the clinician produced a sustained vowel or a brief sentence. Following this pairing of tactile and auditory cues, he was instructed to put his fingers on his own larynx and to attempt to phonate. It took nearly four months of practice for Jim to achieve consistent control over phonation. After this extensive practice, he could produce only "I," "Oh," "Ah," and "Hi" on command. Attempts to stimulate him to combine phonation with speech were unsuccessful. Although Jim had improved from his earlier state of "speechlessness" after four months of treatment, his best efforts at verbal communication consisted of intermittent, painstaking vocalizations accompanied by gross movements of the mandible and tongue.

Other Modalities. In conjunction with his gestural, phonatory, and articulatory training Jim worked on a variety of metalinguistic tasks to improve his auditory comprehension, reading, and writing. His auditory comprehension improved rapidly. After four months of treatment, he was able to understand what was said in most daily situations. He could read single high frequency words. He improved his ability to copy material with his left hand but did not develop spontaneous writing.

Results. Table 10.1 shows Jim's Overall, Gestural, Verbal, and Graphic mean scores on the PICA at the start of treatment (4 months postonset) and throughout his treatment course. Percentile rankings, based on norms for bilaterally damaged subjects (Porch, 1971) are also provided. Table 10.1 shows that Jim improved his Overall, Gestural, and Graphic scores on the PICA from the beginning of treatment to nine months postonset (after 122 treatment sessions), but his PICA Verbal score showed no change in this time period.

Daily treatment results revealed that Jim was improving on those tasks worked on in treatment (e.g., written sentence completion, word and sentence reading), particularly if they did not require speaking. At 9 months postonset Jim still used no speech. He communicated by using a few gestures and a notebook filed with names, phone numbers, letters, drawings, and maps. He tended to refer to this collection of materials as something to "fill in gaps" for his listeners when gestures or pointing failed. This process necessitated a significant amount of guessing and was time consuming.

Family circumstances prevented Jim from continuing his individual treatment at this time. He was discharged but agreed to attend an outpatient communication group. His attendance at group meetings soon became sporadic, and he was totally discharged from any kind of treatment.

Augmentative Communication

After nearly two years without treatment (35 months postonset), Jim was readmitted to the VA hospital. The purpose of this admission was to prepare Jim to enter a vocational training program. Since communication skills were vital to work success, he was reevaluated by speech pathology. The PICA was readministered (see Table 10.1). Results revealed slight improvements in PICA scores in comparison to results two years earlier, but these gains were not reflected in any meaningful changes in Jim's functional communication status. He still communicated with a limited repertoire of gestures, his notebook, and a few monosyllabic utterances he had acquired on his own.

Jim spent four months in the hospital while participating in a vocational rehabilitation program funded by the state of Missouri. Throughout this period he attended group speech and language therapy sessions. His ADL skills improved sufficiently to be discharged to a living situation connected with a closed-workshop setting. At this point, it appeared that Jim would not develop functional verbal communication, and that his use of gestural, notebook, and limited verbal expression would be inadequate in an independent living situation. A decision was made to try another approach that might provide him with a more effective communication system.

The Handi-Voice. At 44 months postonset, and now as an outpatient, Jim was reenrolled in the VAMC Speech and Language Program. He was introduced to the Handi-Voice 110 (H-V). This instrument is one of a number of augmentative communication systems for the speech handicapped. It is a portable, battery operated unit that produces synthesized speech. The device is operated by depressing one of 128 cells systematically arranged on a pressure sensitive grid. It contains a 473-item fixed vocabulary consisting of words, phonemes, syllables, letters, and phrases and can be programmed to produce a variety of synthesized speech signals.

Jim appeared to be an excellent candidate for an augmentative device. His visual motor sequencing skills were sufficiently adequate that he could use the instrument quickly and accurately. His reading had improved and he could recognize the vocabulary items on the grid. Although he had no verbal communication, his aphasic deficits had sufficiently resolved so that he might become a functional communicator if provided with a functional output modality. Finally, he was extremely enthusiastic about the possibility of learning to use the H-V.

Training with the Handi-Voice

For the next seven months Jim received two and one half hours of daily instruction using the H-V. Initially he was instructed in the use of the basic functions of the instrument (e.g., the talk and clear cells) and how to select items from the four vocabulary levels of the instrument. Initial practice began with words and phrases having high personal utility to Jim to permit him to express feelings, greetings, and to respond to yes-no questions. He was taught to program phoneme sequences to produce his name, names of family members, and others. In addition, he was introduced to the level 4 vocabulary phrases of the machine such as "I am" ("I have," "I'd like").

Vocabulary Training. Training in the use of the H-V vocabulary followed the steps outlined in Table 10.2.

Vocabulary Expansion. Nouns occupy the first three levels of the H-V. Verbs are included in levels 1 and 2. Level 2 also contains numbers and concepts such as time, months, and seasons. Level 4 contains useful phrases (e.g., "I have") and word endings (e.g., *ed, ing, -s*). Jim was instructed how to chain phrases (level 4) with verbs (levels 1 or 2) and verb endings (level 4). For example, the programming of the sentence "I am eating" would necessitate activation of appropriate cells on level 4 (I am), level 2 (eat), and level 4 (*ing*) and depression of the talk cell. Nouns from the various levels of the instrument were arranged on

TABLE 10.2
Sequence of Training Steps for Handi-Voice Vocabulary

Step 1.	Identify vocabulary item on H-V in terms of location on grid and level.
Step 2.	Use selected vocabulary item in sentence completion and/or picture identification task.
Step 3.	Use item in conversation, story retelling, or role play activity
Step 4.	Practice vocabulary item in presence of clinician.
	Write independently the response for each vocabulary item using a sentence level and noting location.
	Enter vocabulary items in book.
	Practice programming items in book on H-V in the evening.

the grid according to categories (e.g., food, clothing, body parts) to facilitate learning.

Sentence Programming. Since the reason for using the H-V was to provide Jim with a means of communicating in daily life, a substantial amount of time was spent on sentence programming. This training involved use of the instrument's memory to program, to store, and to retrieve sentences. Jim had attempted to produce sentences in early training with the device, but these had consisted primarily of short telegraphic messages. This phase of treatment was designed to encourage him to program longer, more grammatically complete synthetic utterances.

Table 10.3 summarizes the task sequence used in developing sentence structure. Jim was presented action pictures one at a time. First, he was instructed to write a sentence response. Next he practiced programming and reproducing the sentence on the H-V. Responses were requested in written form first to assist Jim in using appropriate word order. The reason that this procedure could be followed was that Jim had improved his speed and accuracy in writing with his left hand secondary to his practice with the H-V. He was able to write to dictation and ultimately learned to write words and phrases from the H-V vocabulary spontaneously.

TABLE 10.3
Sequence of Training Steps for Sentence Programming

Clinician presents action picture (e.g., A boy eating cake)
Patient:

Step 1.	Examines stimulus picture.
Step 2.	Copies sentence describing picture with single word missing (e.g., The boy is _____ cake).
Step 3.	Determines missing word and programs this word on the H-V.
Step 4.	Programs entire sentence on H-V.
Step 5.	Listens to H-V programmed signal.
Step 6.	Checks for accuracy of missing target item by lifting tab concealing target word on stimulus sentence.
Step 7.	If missing word was produced correctly, reprograms sentence and listens again.

If incorrect, begins entire sequence again.

After almost 7 months of training (52 months postonset) with the H-V, the PICA was readministered (see Table 10.1). In this test Jim was permitted to use the H-V to respond to the verbal subtests of the PICA. Results show that his PICA Verbal scores increased from the 20th to the 48th percentile, verifying the effects of H-V training and its partial circumvention of his severe motor programming disorder. Other PICA modality scores remained unchanged from the prior evaluation, but Jim did show a slight increase in his Overall PICA score as a consequence of his improvement on the PICA Verbals.

At this point his communication involved synthetic speech, gestures, use of his communication book, writing, and a combination of these endeavors. When familiar topics were discussed. Jim communicated proficiently with the H-V, but when less familiar topics were involved the burden of communication fell upon the listener. A typical conversational sequence is shown below:

Jim: Hi, Dr. _____, how are you?
Clinician: Fine, Jim, how are you?

Jim: I'm fine and I'm ready to work.
Clinician: Great Jim, let's get started.
Jim: I'm tired (sheepish grin, eyebrows raised).
Clinician: Oh no you don't. I've heard that one before.
Jim: Angry. I have angry.
Clinician: Angry? About what?
Jim: Cardinals (thumb pointing down), bad.
Clinician: You mean they (a baseball team) lost again?
Jim: No (shaking head).
Clinician: Did they make a poor trade?
Jim: Yes (looking relieved), bad.

Return of Speech

As he prepared for discharge, Jim continued to work on perfecting his use of the augmentative system. At the end of one of his afternoon treatment sessions, the clinician encouraged him to count out loud (a practice periodically tried but usually resulting in a perseverative "uh" accompanied by gross movements of the articulators). Surprisingly, he responded in a deep, resonant voice and counted from 1 to 10. Sensing that something significant had occurred, the clinician and the patient moved to an adjacent room and videotaped what was to follow. Jim counted with the clinician in unison, and continued to count intelligibly when the clinician withdrew from participation. He responded to simple questions requiring numerical answers (e.g., How many days in a week?). He repeated his first name after the clinician, and after a short rest spontaneously said "Jim" using perfect articulation. He was able to use greetings such as "Hi," "Bye," and "How are you?" and gave accurate "yes" and "no" replies to a variety of questions. When asked what he thought of the sound of his voice, he said "Good" and prolonged the vowel for emphasis. Perhaps in response to the emotion of the situation he spontaneously said "beer" while gesturing with a drinking motion.

All of the aforementioned utterances were produced within a 40-minute period after the surprising return of speech. By 4:30 on the same day he had produced 97 different words and phrases either spontaneously, in sentence completion tasks, or imitatively. He seemed to be able to monitor his sudden return of speech. The articulation errors he did make were usually phoneme substitutions (e.g., "bork" for "fork"), anticipatory errors, or misarticulated sound blends. He corrected many of these with little effort.

In the next few days he produced more than 200 new words. The range of his vocabulary was surprisingly broad. For example, when asked about his favorite music, he replied "Play music? Barbra Streis-

and, John Denver, Rocky Mountain High." When asked about the return of speech by fellow group patients, he counted backwards from ten to one and enthusiastically said "Blast off."

The Handi-Voice: A New Role. It was thought that practice with the H-V had facilitated Jim's improved writing. Continued practice using the augmentative system now served to cue production of spoken responses. When he was unable to produce a verbal response, he located the desired item on the instrument grid, listened to the synthetic speech representation, and produced the verbal response. For the next few months treatment efforts were directed toward use of the device in combination with verbal expression.

Three weeks after his speech returned Jim's spoken vocabulary count rose to more than 400 words. In another week he had mastered more than 500 words. He could now generate complete sentences to describe action pictures. For example, in response to the question "Who is playing ball?" he replied, "The boy is playing ball." What had taken several months to achieve with the H-V, was now being accomplished at a much more rapid rate.

Results. Three months after the return of his speech and treatment emphasizing use of the H-V in conjunction with speech (55½ months postonset), the PICA was readministered. This time Jim was not allowed to use the H-V. Table 10.1 shows that PICA Verbal scores increased 14 percentile points from his prior test on which he used the H-V only. Jim could now respond relevantly to all the PICA Verbal subtests. Repetition on the PICA was flawless; naming and sentence completion responses were accurate, delayed, or self-corrected; and sentence formulation was agrammatic and telegraphic.

Follow-up

At approximately 55½ months postonset, now communicating verbally, Jim moved into an apartment designed for handicapped individuals. He continued to receive outpatient speech and language treatment at the VA Medical Center. PICA testing carried out at five years postonset (60 months) showed additional improvement in Verbal scores. His test performance was distinguished by a reduction of self-corrections and improved ability to produce complete sentences on PICA subtest I from his prior PICA testing. On this test (55½ postonset), Jim had improved 25 percentile points on the PICA Graphics. This was primarily the results of improved accuracy in writing to dictation.

At five years postonset Jim was discharged from formal treatment. He began a job operating a newsstand at a nearby medical center. He communicated on the job and with his friends using speech, the H-V, writing, gesturing, and his communication notebook. His verbal language remained telegraphic and agrammatic.

Final Outcome

Jim received another follow-up evaluation at nine years postonset (107.0 months). Sometime between this point and his dismissal from formal treatment, he discarded the augmentative device and informed the VA staff that he no longer needed it. He continues to live independently in his apartment, to operate the newsstand, and to visit the VA occasionally for social interaction with the staff. His verbal communication is telegraphic, requiring a significant amount of interpretation by his listeners, but his communication is functional.

The PICA was administered (see Table 10.1). Modest reductions in scores were evidenced in all modalities and in the Overall PICA mean, but this was not totally unexpected given the length of time elapsed between this evaluation and cessation of treatment. The good news was that Jim was communicating, and he was communicating verbally. A transcription of his conversation with the clinician and description of the "Cookie Theft" picture from the *Boston Diagnostic Aphasia Exam* (Goodglass & Kaplan, 1972) illustrates his skill.

Clinician: Tell me what you've been doing.
Jim: Work—paperboy
Clinician: About how many papers do you sell each day?
Jim: 21 (pause) thousand. No 21.
Clinician: When do you get up in the morning?
Jim: 6:30
Clinician: And when do you finish?
Jim: 10 0'clock (pause) hungry!
Clinician: Where are you living these days?
Jim: Forrest Park, handicapped apartments—no girls!

Cookie Theft Description
Man, boy falling. Boy, woman, girl falling down. Cookies bad. Mrs. dripping water. Burning? Weird.

Jim's Overall PICA scores throughout treatment are graphed in Figure 10.1. Figure 10.2 shows PICA modality scores for the same time period. These data indicate that most of his recovery occurred between 52 and 60 months postonset. When he began to use the H-V, his PICA Verbal scores improved (see Figure 10.2), first, when allowed to use the H-V in taking the PICA, and second, when his speech returned and treatment emphasized H-V and speech. Although Jim did improve his

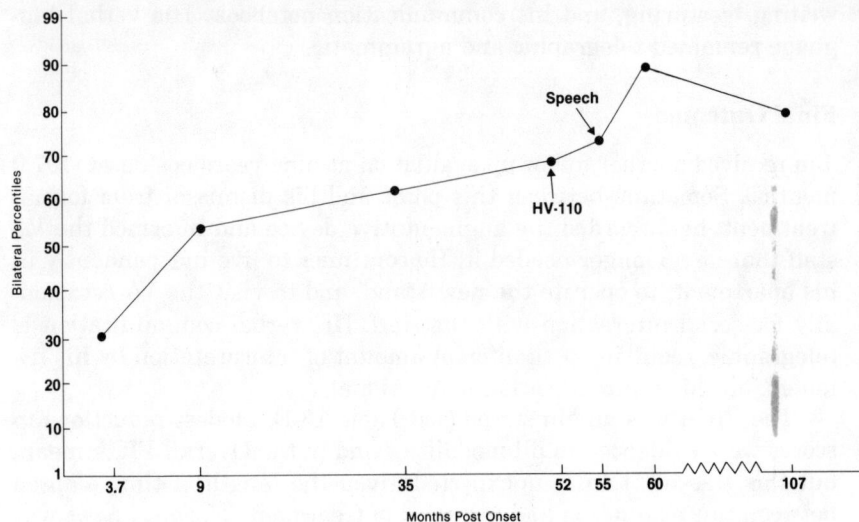

Figure 10.1 Overall percentile rankings for Jim (bilateral norms) on the PICA throughout the treatment course.

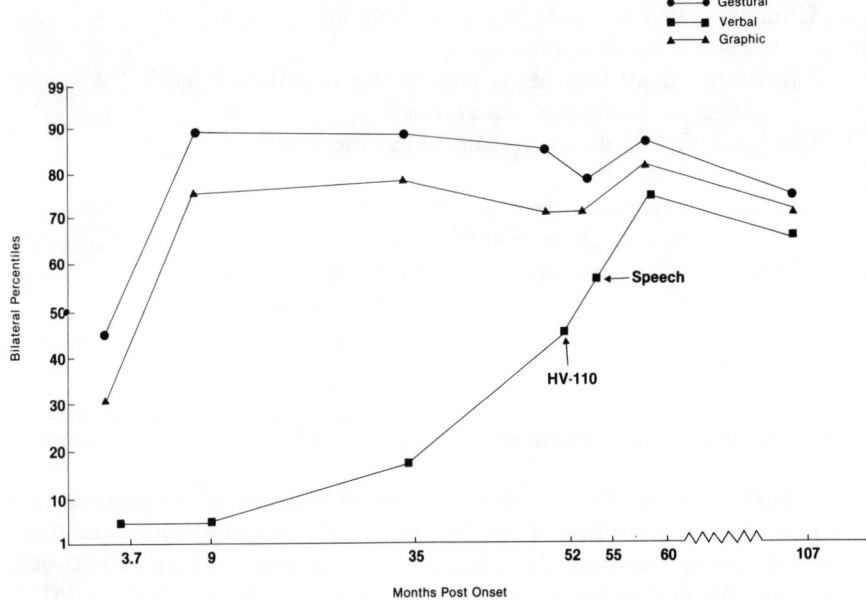

Figure 10.2 Gestural, Verbal, and Graphic modality percentiles for Jim (bilateral norms) on the PICA throughout the course of treatment.

PICA Graphics with treatment, changes were limited and primarily involved better writing to dictation. They had little functional value for Jim.

NATURE OF THE SPEECH DISORDER

A retrospective analysis of Jim's recovery suggests that he had two distinctively different communication deficits: a loss of the capacity of speech, which surprisingly returned at four and one half years postonset, and a Broca's type of aphasia. The characteristics of his aphasia could not really be ascertained until he had acquired sufficient skill with the augmentative device (generating telegraphic sentences) and later, reacquired speech. Abilities in other language modalities (e.g., gesturing and writing), however, seemed to plateau at nine months postonset and support the notion that he had two communication deficits.

Initially, Jim's lack of speech was attributed to a severe apraxia of speech associated with a severe Broca's aphasia. However, radiological evidence as well as the nature of his articulation following the return of speech did not support diagnosis of a primary, efferent apraxia disturbing motor programming functions. While Jim evidenced some laborious, struggling articulation movements the first day speech returned, these problems were short-lived. He quickly began to correct his errors and to reflect an articulatory pattern within the confines of his telegraphic speaking style that was relatively normal and at times quite animated. Thus, a motor programming deficit such as apraxia of speech (Darley, Aronson, & Brown, 1975) does not explain Jim's speechlessness.

Mutism refers to a total or near total loss of speech and phonation. Mutism is not uncommon during postcoma recovery following closed head injury, but it usually does not persist unless associated with a permanent vegetative state (Levin, Benton, & Grossman, 1982). Akinetic mutism (Plum & Posner, 1980) is a form of the disorder associated with lesions that interfere with reticular-cortical or limbic cortical integration, but spare cortical spinal tracts. Akinetic mutism is also associated with diffuse cerebral injury as well as lacunar infarcts (Geschwind, 1964). However, akinetic mutism usually resolves within several months postcoma. Jim's speech recovery did not correspond to cases of mutism or akinetic mutism.

The rapid return of Jim's speech might also suggest a functional component. Jim, similar to patients with vascular lesions, presented an orderliness in his error patterns that differs from that of individuals attempting to "simulate" aphasia (Porec & Porch, 1977). Specifically, phoneme reapproaches, anticipatory substitutions, increasing difficulty with the length of utterances, and so forth, represented a qualitatively typical reestablishment of phoneme programming and/or selection skills compressed into a late but very brief time frame. Also, it is probably safe to assume that Jim was not malingering for five years.

Following the return of speech, the characteristics of Jim's verbal output may fit Martin's (1974) description of phonological impairment in aphasia or Canter's (1969) secondary (afferent) verbal apraxia. In both instances, disruption of phonological selection and sequencing is viewed as a language-based disorder. However, neither classification can account for a relatively mute condition lasting four and one half years. And, of course, the more intriguing question still remains: Why did Jim's speech return?

Inferences Concerning the Return of Speech

Disconnection. Geschwind (1972) popularized the notion of disconnection as an explanation for loss of specific cortical function; and Levin et al. (1982) have associated limb apraxias in severe closed head injury with intrahemisphere disconnection. Within a disconnection explanation, Jim's sudden return of speech may indicate that Broca's area (which according to CT interpretations was not contained within the boundaries of the lesion per se) may have retained its programming capacity but was isolated from posterior association areas. However, Buckingham (1979) has pointed out that, similar to the specific deficits of tactile naming and limb apraxia, the classical disconnection theory cannot account for total mutism, but only for an inability to speak after verbal command.

Mohr (1980) has suggested that damaged tissue in the dominant hemisphere surrounding Broca's area may interfere with the physiological effort required in the speech act itself. Perhaps Jim's speechlessness was due to an inability to gather the physiological momentum required for overt verbal expression. This leads us to the consideration of the potential facilitative effects of the use of synthetic speech and its role in reestablishing what may be termed within Mohr's (1980) construct as "physiological momentum."

Facilitation. It is intriguing that Jim's speech returned following months of intensive training on a speech synthesizer. Luria's (1970) notion of "intersystemic reorganization" is frequently associated with the facilitative efforts of nonspeech modalities on verbal expression (Collins, Wertz, & Rosenbek, 1976). Gesture (Skelly, 1979) and melodic intonation therapy (Helm, 1976) are commonly used as facilitative devices. Similarly, "deblocking" (Weigl & Bierwisch, 1970) takes advantage of more intact modalities to stimulate use of less intact modalities.

If the H-V was influential in facilitating or deblocking the return of the client's speech, its role has relevance to the much discussed relationship between language and motor programming and the parallel arguments of Darley et al. (1975) and Martin (1974). The H-V may have directly facilitated speech because it stimulated subvocal or implicit rehearsal of the phonetic patterns that the patient associated with the phonemic characteristics of synthetic speech. From a more divergent point of view, and one which relates to Mohr's (1980) comments on the synergistic relationship of language and motor programming functions, the H-V may have enabled Jim to select, sequence, and encode elements of language into a covert, comprehensible form. In turn, this process may have encouraged him to use his residual language skills. Eventually, the increased use of the language system may have achieved enough "inertia" or momentum to activate a dormant yet relatively intact motor programming system. Similarly, Feyersen (1982) describes a model of nonverbal motor planning in which movements occurring in response to commands (e.g., confrontation to speak) are not comparable to "naturally released signals." Intensive use of the H-V could have elicited natural, less confrontative commands to stimulate implicit rehearsal of articulation patterns, eventually producing overt speech.

Augmentative Devices

Some comments about the use of augmentative systems with language impaired individuals are warranted. Hagen, Parker, and Brink (1973) have emphasized that the success of these systems depends on the interaction of mechanical and cognitive/linguistic variables and the response of the members of the environment to the patient's use of the system. Beukelman and Yorkston (1980) point out the need to evaluate the listener's acceptance of an augmentative system, and that this acceptance, coupled with the user's confidence in the system, are the essential ingredients of success.

Most clinicians have treated patients who had the ability to use augmentative communication systems such as gesture and/or synthetic speech devices but did not develop competence with the systems because they insisted on talking. While most clinicians have accepted the need to work on "communication" instead of talking (Holland, 1977), it has not been determined whether our patients share this viewpoint. Jim was no exception. It was disappointing that he did not use gestures learned in the clinic spontaneously. He preferred to use static forms of communication such as words and pictures in his notebook despite the fact that these were less efficient than his gestural communication. Even though he became proficient in using the augmentative system, he resorted to less efficient communicative modes in difficult situations.

When his speech finally returned, Jim used the Handi-Voice to cue himself for word and phrase productions, but as soon as his capacity for spoken language increased, he discarded the augmentative device, even as a back-up system. Perhaps he made the right choice? His return of speech, however, underscores the point that augmentative systems are truly augmentative. Despite our clinical interests in having the patient use multiple systems (gesture, writing, notebook, and synthetic speech) for flexibility, back-up, or self-cuing, once the patient has decided that he no longer needs an assistive device, he resorts to the form of communication that truly distinguishes man from lower forms.

Final Comment

Most likely, we will never fully understand why speech returned to Jim. Nevertheless, all of us who treated and know this young man believe that our efforts over the years made it possible for Jim to live and communicate as an independent, functioning member of society. This clinician feels most fortunate to have worked and shared in this experience.

ACKNOWLEDGMENT

I would like to express appreciation to Dr. Dee Jay Hubbard for his assistance and to acknowledge the cooperation of the Veterans Administration.

REFERENCES

Beukelman, D., & Yorkston, D. (1980). Nonvocal communication: Performance evaluation. *Archives of Physical Medicine and Rehabilitation, 61,* 272–275.

Buckingham, H.W. (1979). Explanation in apraxia with consequences for the concept of apraxia of speech. *Brain and Language, 8,* 202–226.

Canter, G.J. (1969, November). *The influence of primary and secondary verbal apraxia in output disturbances in aphasic syndromes.* Paper presented at the Annual Convention of the American Speech Hearing Association, Chicago.

Collins, M., Wertz, R.T., & Rosenbek, J.C. (1976, November). *Intersystemic reorganization for apraxia of speech.* Paper presented at the Annual Convention of the American Speech Hearing Association, Houston.

Darley, F.L., Aronson, A.F., & Brown, J.P. (1975). *Motor speech disorders.* Philadelphia: W.B. Sanders.

Feyersen, P.S.X. (1982). Nonverbal communication and aphasia: A review. *Brain and Language, 16,* 213–236.

Geschwind, N. (1964). Nonaphasic disorders of speech. *International Journal of Neurology, 4,* 207–214.

Geschwind, N. (1972). Language and the brain. *Scientific American, 226,* 76–83.

Goodglass, H., & Kaplan, E. (1972). *The assessment of aphasia and related disorders.* Philadelphia: Lee and Febiger.

Hagen, C., Parker, W., & Brink, J. (1973). Nonverbal communication: An alternate mode of communication for the child with severe cerebral palsy. *Journal of Speech and Hearing Disorders, 38,* 448–455.

Helm, N. (1976, November). *Assessing candidacy for melodic intonation therapy*. Paper presented at the Annual Convention of the American Speech and Hearing Association, Houston.

Holland, A.L. (1977). Some practical considerations in aphasia rehabilitation. In H. Sullivan and M. Kommers (Eds.), *Rationale for adult aphasia therapy*. Omaha: University of Nebraska Medical Center.

Levin, H., Benton, A., & Grossman, R. (1982). *Neurobehavioral consequences of closed head injury*. New York: Oxford University Press.

Luria, A.R. (1970). *Traumatic aphasia*. The Hague, Netherlands: Mouton.

Martin. A.I. (1974). Some objections to the term apraxia of speech. *Journal of Speech and Hearing Disorders, 39,* 53–64.

Mohr, J.P. (1980). Revision of Broca's aphasia and the syndrome of Broca's area infarction and its implications on aphasia theory. In R.H. Brookshire (Ed.), *Clinical Aphasiology Conference Proceedings*. Minneapolis: BRK Publishers.

Plum, F., & Posner, J. (1980). *The diagnosis of stupor and coma*. Philadelphia: F.A. Davis Company.

Porch, B.E. (1971). *The Porch Index of Communicative Ability*. Palo Alto, CA: Consulting Psychologists Press.

Porec, J., & Porch, B. (1971). The behavioral characteristics of "simulated" aphasia. In R.H. Brookshire (Ed.), *Clinical Aphasiology Conference Proceedings*. Minneapolis: BRK Publishers.

Skelly, M. (1979). *American Indian gestural code*. New York: Elsevier North Holland.

Weigl, E., & Bierwisch, M. (1970). Neuropsychology and linguistics: Topics of common research. *Foundations of Language, 6,* 1–18.

CHAPTER 11
The Center for Independent Living: A Case Study
Cheri L. Florance and William F. Conway

> *Florance (a speech-language pathologist) and Conway (a physician) direct a unique contemporary program for the comprehensive medical management and rehabilitation of geriatric persons. The Center for Independent Living (CIL) of Columbus, Ohio is an interdisciplinary unit having as its primary goal the maintaining of patient automony and independence. Improvement of cognitive and communicative abilities are the responsibilities of all members of the interdisciplinary team. The authors describe the evaluation and treatment of a 76-year-old aphasic stroke victim within the CIL.*

1. How do the evaluational procedures employed by the CIL differ from those normally employed with aphasic persons? What information from CIL evaluations can be used to plan treatment? To render a prognosis? Does the evaluation process itself have any therapeutic value?
2. What part do significant others, occupational therapists, and other interdisciplinary team members play in the cognitive and communicative rehabilitation of the patient?
3. Florance and Conway suggest that improvement in the patient's communication will prompt improvement in other areas (e.g., ADLs, coping, and compliance) as well. How is this accomplished? How are results measured?

INTRODUCTION

We experience three biological units within our life: growth and development, maturation, and senescence. In senescence we are increasingly vulnerable to disease and experience decreased vitality as our body organs undergo the decline process. Most aphasic patients are experiencing the process of senescence. To design appropriate rehabilitation for these patients, we must see them within biological as well as medical contexts.

A second condition is the impact of a stroke on the patient and his family. One day patients may be in complete control of their activities. Suddenly, without warning or an opportunity to prepare emotionally, they may awaken in the hospital unable to feed themselves, remember, talk, or think clearly. To manage these unexpected life changes, the patient needs to draw upon the internal coping and defense mechanisms that develop over one's lifetime. Individuals with a wide repertoire of these mechanisms cope when they can, are open to change, and defend when they must. This allows them to protect the status quo. Persons without these mechanisms to tap may fragment and lose their emotional equilibrium. In such instances, the patient may illustrate confusion, inappropriate speech and language, poor memory, lack of problem solving ability, and be unable to separate and organize information.

Finally, as human beings, we tend to interact within our species primarily through verbal communication. This interchange requires a speaker and a listener. When one of these dyad members is an impaired aphasic stroke victim, it will affect the behavior of the other. Therefore, to understand clearly the problems faced by aphasic persons, we need to view these patients within their particular community.

CENTER FOR INDEPENDENT LIVING (CIL)

In an effort to develop a rehabilitation unit capable of addressing the aforementioned issues, the Center for Independent Living (CIL) was designed to provide specialized, comprehensive, medical, and rehabilitative services. In the CIL, professional disciplines are intertwined so that the patient is seen as more than a subspecialty and as an individual within his own life context. The transdisciplinary team works together to develop appropriate recommendations and treatment plans. More important, the team strives to devise and implement treatment strategies which have, as a primary goal, maintaining patient autonomy and functional performance levels adequate for independent living. This goal unites the team so that the patient receives a singular service strengthened by multiple modalities.

This case report documents the evaluation, treatment, and progress of a 76-year-old woman who suffered a stroke and became aphasic.

THE CASE: MS. ROYER

Ms. Royer was referred to the CIL by her friend, Ms. Mapes, with whom she had been living following hospital discharge. According to Ms. Mapes, Ms. Royer was despondent, confused, and disoriented during her hospitalization. She appeared to have poor comprehension, reasoning, and speech. On the advice of her physician and the hospital social worker, she sold her home and belongings, gave power of attorney over her affairs and finances to Ms. Mapes' son, and planned for a nursing home admission. At the time of discharge, however, no nursing home beds were available, and Ms. Mapes agreed to care for her while a placement was sought.

While living in Ms. Mapes' guest room, Ms. Royer became increasingly withdrawn and noncommunicative and had little appetite and difficulty sleeping. She became very demanding of Ms. Mapes, insisting that she not be left alone in the house. Because Ms. Mapes felt that Ms. Royer should be further evaluated, she discussed the possibility of a CIL evaluation with her. Ms. Royer reluctantly agreed to make the appointment, reportedly only because one of her former high school students worked at the CIL.

Medical History

Past medical history was obtained from records at St. Anthony Hospital. Ms. Royer had life-long hypertension controlled by the use of a diuretic. In October 1983, she began to have episodes of dizziness and fainting. She was admitted to the hospital for evaluation of her apparent syncope. While in the hospital, an EKG revealed the onset of atrial fibrillation. The fibrillation had a rapid ventricular response, and she was subsequently digitalized, She responded well to digitalization, and her ventricular rate became controlled. However, her rhythm did not convert to sinus. She was subsequently discharged. Approximately three weeks after discharge, she again noted the onset of fainting episodes. These became more frequent and were associated with numbness and tingling, as well as with difficulties in communication. She was readmitted to the hospital for evaluation of these acute episodes. While in the hospital, her ventricular rate remained controlled. She underwent carotid endarterectomy. Following the endarterectomy, she suffered a stroke with resulting right hemiplegia and communication deficits. A CT scan of the head revealed an infarction of the left hemisphere. Over a period of four days, her hemiplegia resolved totally, but the communication problems persisted.

Physical Examination

Examination revealed a pleasant white female who appeared somewhat younger than her stated age of 75. She was of average weight with minimal to moderate wrinkling. Vital signs on examination were blood pressure 150/90, pulse 80 and irregular, respiration 16. The head and face were symmetric at rest. The sclera were clear. There was a cataract noted on the left eye. Extraocular movements were intact. There was a large amount of cerumen in the left ear. Tympanic membranes were pearly gray with good reflex. The mouth was edentulous with pink mucous membranes. The uvula was symmetric at rest and on movement. The neck was supple. Carotid pulses were strong bilaterally. No masses or enlarged lymph nodes were noted in the neck. Inspection of the thorax revealed a slightly increased AP diameter. Percussion of the thorax revealed resonance throughout. On auscultation, breath sounds were vesicular, with a slightly long expiration. No adventitia was noted. The PMI was in the fifth intercostal space, slightly displaced to the left of the midclavicular line. Cardiac rhythm was grossly irregular. There were no gallops or murmurs. The breasts were symmetric, atrophic without masses. The abdomen was slightly protuberant and soft. Bowel sounds were active and present. Percussion of the abdomen revealed tympany throughout. No tenderness or rebound tenderness was noted on lighted palpation. On deep palpation no masses or organomegaly were noted. The genitals were atrophic. There were no masses in the rectum. The stool was normal. Muscle tone was good in all extremities. There was no spasticity. There were no flexion contractures. Reflexes were equal and symmetric. Cranial nerves appeared intact. The feet were cold with diffuse loss of hair and thickening of the nails. The pulses were strong bilaterally.

Laboratory Findings

Chest x-ray in October, 1983, revealed minimal cardiomegaly. EKG showed atrial fibrillation with controlled ventricular responses. White blood count was 4.6; Hemaglobin 40; MCV 98; MCH 31.8; MCHC 32.6; Glucose was 98; BUN 14; uric acid 3.6; calcium 86; total protein 6.1; albumin 3.2; sodium 139; potassium 4.3; and chloride 104. The Snellen visual test revealed vision in the left eye was 20/200, and vision in the right eye was 20/100. CT scan of the head revealed an infarction of the left hemisphere.

ASSESSMENT OF SUPPORT SYSTEMS

During administration of *The Independent Living Self-Assessment* (Florance, 1984), Ms. Royer indicated she was estranged from her family. Although she reported that several of her nieces and nephews came to visit her, she felt that they were merely trying to calculate what they might inherit and she felt no emotional support from them. She stated that she was too "old, sick, and feeble-minded" to manage on her own. She hated the idea of living in a "public place" but had no other solution.

On the *Family Administered Home Assessment* (Florance, 1984), Ms. Mapes reported that before Ms. Royer had her stroke she had a large social network. She played the organ at her church, participated in a variety of social clubs, and served as a French lecturer at a local university. She traveled extensively out of the state, and frequently out of the country. She was seen as a pillar of her community, having taught in the same school system for over 40 years. She was an avid reader and continued to thrive on education, often enrolling in both adult education and academic courses.

OCCUPATIONAL THERAPY EVALUATION

Self-Care

This patient was able to complete all self-care and grooming tasks adequately. Her upper extremity muscle strength and active range of motion were adequate for dressing, bathing, and grooming needs. She was able to ambulate and transfer adequately to use the bathroom facilities. She reported that she felt tired and as though there were no need to bother with her appearance.

Financial Management

Ms. Royer could determine an appropriate budget for planning a dinner party and estimate the cash value of the needed groceries. She was able to balance a simulated checkbook, read bills, and write appropriate checks for payment. She appeared to compensate for her language impairment by copying the company's name and the amount of the bill on the check. She was unable to fill in the check accurately from verbal dictation. She was able to manage withdrawal and deposit transactions in the simulation bank at the teller station. She was easily taught to use the Handibank Machine. She indicated that she would much prefer to use the Handibank as she would not need to communicate verbally.

Shopping, Meal Planning and Preparation

When attempting to make a sample grocery list, the patient was unable to list the items verbally or in writing. In both cases, she made off-target attempts at a variety of words until she became angry and gave up. However, she was able to circle items from a written list of food groups. In the simulation grocery store, she easily identified the items which were appropriate for her preplanned dinner party meal. At the checkout counter, she reacted appropriately to an error made by the "cashier" before paying her bill and then made proper payment.

Home Safety

The patient was asked to role play emergency management of fire, theft, and medical crises. She attempted to participate but quickly became frustrated due to her poor communicative ability and refused to continue the task. She was easily trained to use the emergency management equipment, however, and she indicated that she felt capable of staying at home with these supplemental devices to aid her in calling for help. She located the numbers for police, fire, the emergency squad, and her physician in the telephone book and dialed the numbers appropriately. However, she refused to converse on the phone, indicating that she could not talk adequately. She reaffirmed that since her stroke she had been quite fearful of being left alone. She indicated that although she felt guilty about it, she had pleaded with Ms. Mapes to make sure someone was always with her.

Transportation Evaluation

Ms. Royer was tested at the Drivers' Simulation Center using the simulation films "Basic Training" and "Control Driving" with the following results:

Basic Training Tasks	Correct Responses	Controlled Driving Tasks	Correct Responses
Signaling	78%	Signaling	71%
Steering	80%	Steering	80%
Braking	84%	Braking	69%
Speeding	89%	Speeding	75%
Acceleration	78%	Acceleration	82%

Ms. Royer was able to locate phone numbers to contact cab companies but was unable to communicate her request for services adequately. She was able to indicate appropriate routes on a map for traveling to various community locations.

COMMUNICATION

On the Adult Communication Analysis (ACA) (Florance, 1981), speech samples were collected in the home and in the clinic, with test scores as follows:

	Clinic	Home
Communicative Services	40%	68%
Intelligibilty	0%	0%
Appropriateness	40%	68%
Efficiency	0%	0%
Comprehension	40%	68%
Mean Length of Utterance	3.4	2.6

Each of her communication attempts contained multiple off-target productions of single words. She often became frustrated by these errors and refused to continue her communicative attempts. When she did complete a speech act adequately enough for the listener to understand, her response was appropriate, suggesting that she understood the context of the conversation.

The *Analysis of Interaction Dynamics* (AID) (Florance, 1984) is a scale designed to score the patient's ability to maintain and further a conversation. Ms. Royer's test scores were severely impaired in all parameters including relationship dynamics, peer interaction, conversational responsibility, attending behavior, clinical and nonclinical interaction, initiating, elaboration, semantic content, positive/negative focus, and conversational directionality.

On the *Family Interaction Analysis* (FIA) (Florance, 1981), the clinician tabulates those behaviors exhibited by the significant other, before and after the patient's communicative attempts. For Ms. Royer the following levels of communicative success were obtained: (1) paraphrasing content, 80%; (2) reflecting feeling, 80%; (3) minimal encouragers, 75%; (4) open questions, 50%; and (5) closed questions, 20%.

On the *Porch Index of Communicative Ability* (PICA) (Porch, 1967), Ms.Royer had an Overall Gestural score of 14.85 and an Overall Verbal score of 13.18. She rejected all of the Graphic subtests except copying tasks E and F which she performed correctly. On the *Oral-Verbal Apraxia Battery* (Florance, 1975), her test performance was within normal limits on the oral subtests. However, on verbal subtests her scores were markedly impaired.

COPING AND COMPLIANCE ASSESSMENT (CCA)

The *Coping and Compliance Assessment* (Florance, 1982) is a statistical analysis of the patient's coping and defense repertoire and personality profile derived from psychometric scales. Test results are as follows:

Coping

Psychiatric Disease. The patient presented a profile suggestive of clinical depression. There were no data to support the existence of any other psychiatric diseases. The disorders screened included hypochondriasis, hysteria, sociopathy, male/female paranoia, obsessive-compulsive tendencies, schizophrenia, hypomania, and introversion.

Coping and Defense Repertoire. Nine of Ms. Royer's coping and defense mechanisms were within normal limits, and four were found to be severely impaired. The impaired dyads involved the primary cognitive coping-defense mechanisms, which could result in impaired judgment, reasoning, and problem solving.

Her coping and defense strengths were related to management of her feelings. She appeared able to evaluate the needs of others with sensitivity and to control her emotions in socially tolerated ways. She was not preoccupied with the possibility that others would maltreat her.

Sense of Well-Being. The patient presented with a severe impairment in her sense of well-being, suggesting an undue emphasis on negative life aspects, physical ailments, and personal problems. She had a decreased sense of self-worth and an impaired ability to withstand stress. She presented with increased anxiety and impoverished socialization.

Compliance

Cognition and Problem Solving

A. Coping Defense Repertoire
   This patient presented with a severe impairment in the four primary cognitive coping-defense dyads including:
   1. Objectivity/Isolation: She was unable to distinguish facts from feelings.
   2. Intellectuality/Intellectualization: She was unable to apply abstract ideas in solving problems and develop appropriate solutions.
   3. Logical Analysis/Rationalization: She gave unlikely reasons for past actions and linked implausible chains of events.
   4. Concentration/Denial: She focused on irrelevant aspects of problems and was easily distracted, preventing her from completing tasks.

B. Intellectual Ability

The patient presented with a preference for achievement by independence rather than conformity, indicating a high self-reinforcer personality type. She appeared to have the ability to set goals and plan reasonable and efficient solutions to problems.

Behavior Change Style. Ms. Royer demonstrated a high need for autonomy and internal locus of control, a high tolerance for ambiguity, and an ability to be flexible. She demonstrated the ability to participate in the design and implementation of her own treatment plan. No abnormal scores were found in the areas of responsibility, socialization, self-control or sociopathy.

COGNITION

Prior to her CVA Ms. Royer was administered the *Wechsler Adult Intelligence Scale (WAIS)* (Wechsler, 1955) as part of her involvement in an endarterectomy research program. The WAIS was readministered poststroke to determine any change in her cognitive level. Comparative test scores were as follows:

	Prestroke	Poststroke
Verbal I.Q.	129	119
Performance I.Q.	114	112
Full-scale I.Q.	124	117

APPRAISAL OF PATIENT STATUS

Medical

Ms. Royer's central chronic illness had been hypertension, which was well-controlled with Dyazide. In light of her recent CVA, it will be important to maintain a reasonable control of her blood pressure. However, it is equally important not to achieve a control which is too rigorous. In the senescent patient, it has been well observed that abruptly lowering blood pressures, or tightly controlling blood pressures, results in an increased risk of CVAs as well as encephalopathies, which will acutely affect both communication and cognition. Fibrillation is another risk factor for cerebrovascular accident. Currently well-controlled on Lanoxin, it will be important to maintain a normal ventricular rate and to avoid the formation of an intraventricular thrombus. A trial period of antidepressant medication was recommended. Otherwise, her medical illnesses were well-controlled. On the basis of her medical illnesses alone, she did not require the level of care given in a nursing home.

Occupational Therapy

This patient appeared to have a significant impairment in Activities of Daily Living (ADL). She rejected any attempt to manage her daily needs beyond her personal hygiene. Results of our assessment indicated that when ADL tasks required speaking or writing she failed, but when she was permitted to engage in tasks that required thinking in the absence of speaking, she succeeded. These findings suggested that her reasoning, problem solving, and judgment were adequate for most ADL tasks.

Communication

Ms. Royer manifests a severe communication disorder secondary to apraxia of speech. Spontaneous writing was severely impaired, but comprehension of written and verbal language appeared intact. As a result of her inability to communicate conversationally, she rejected nearly all activities of daily living and chose to live a solitary hermit-type existence with little interaction with other people or seeking of other forms of stimulation. An improvement in her ability to communicate should have a profound impact on her ADLs, human interaction, and coping and compliance behaviors.

Coping and Compliance

This patient's overall profile is one of clinical depression, impaired cognitive, coping, and defense mechanisms, coupled with a poor sense of well-being. Her emotional response to her illness and subsequent speech disorder suggests that she has undergone a marked change in her cognitive abilities. With more opportunities for communicative success, she should be able to manage change readily as long as she participates in the design of her treatment plan. She will then have a data based reality for achieving greater success in her ADLs and independent self-management. Designing an intervention approach which carefully builds upon success should permit her to regain autonomy and permit her to return to her prehospitalization coping and compliance status.

Cognition

Reportedly the patient was confused and disoriented during her hospitalization. At the time of this testing, her standardized test performance was within normal limits for all cognitive parameters. These findings were also supported by her performance in the simulation laboratories suggesting that her basic cognitive function was adequate for independent living without supervision. However, she initially appeared to have problems in the areas of coping and compliance, preventing her from being able to use her cognitive ability for daily self-management.

INTERVENTION STRATEGY

The results of the evaluation suggested that the patient's primary problem was lack of communication success. Because she could not convey her messages successfully, she withdrew from activities of daily living, which over time resulted in an impaired coping and compliance profile. Knowledge of her premorbid functions suggested that prior to her stroke she was managing independently. If in treatment she was able to increase instances of communicative success, rapid changes might be seen in her ability to manage her ADLs and in her coping and compliance profile.

Because Ms. Royer presented a profile suggestive of a high self-reinforcer or one who needs to maintain independence and autonomy, she was enrolled in individual treatment. Her treatment was delivered within a Rogerian format so that she could help determine the appropriate content for the treatment sessions. Her significant other was included in later stages of treatment at her request.

Speech Treatment

As shown in Table 11.1, her speech treatment consisted of six phases. In Phase I, the speech clinician used the interviewing tactics found to be most effective on the *Family Interaction Analysis* (FIA). Within two hours of professional treatment provided on the first two days of treatment, the patient achieved 100% communicative success in the speech clinic with the clinician. In Phase II, the speech clinician continued to use interviewing tactics in a conversational paradigm while training the patient to self-evaluate her own communicative success. Ms. Royer was able to reliably evaluate her own speech responses after one hour of professional training. In Phase III, the patient received counseling from the speech clinician regarding her readiness for change. This counseling paradigm required the patient to elaborate on a more abstract linguistic level than had been required in the previous sessions. Further, the clinician used nondirective Rogerian tactics to selectively reinforce Ms. Royer's use of the coping strategies of objectivity, intellectuality, logical analysis, and concentration. A total of four hours of treatment time was utilized in Phase III, and Ms. Royer mastered ADL activity in the occupational therapy department concomitantly.

In Phase IV, Ms. Mapes was trained to utilize the interviewing tactics at home in patient generated contracts. The patient predetermined the audience, the duration of the conversational sample, the time of the

TABLE 11.1
Speech Pathology Treatment Plan

PHASE	STIMULUS	GOAL	EVALUATOR	LOCATION	COVARIABLES ASSESSMENT	PROFESSIONAL TIME	WEEK
I. Training Target Behavior	Speech Clinician Uses Interview Tactics	100% C.S.	Speech Clinician	Speech Clinic	ACA HLA	2 hrs.	1
II. Independent Self-Management	Speech Clinician Uses Interview Tactics	100% C.S.	Patient	Speech Clinic	ACA HLA	1 hr.	1
III. Transfer to Clincial Environments	Speech Clinician Provides Counseling While Transfer Begins in O.T.	100% C.S.	Speech Clinician	Speech Clinic	ACA HLA	4 hrs.	1 + 2
IV. Transfer to Non-Clincial Environments	Significant Other Uses Interviewing Tactics in Pt. Generated Contracts	100% C.S.	Patient	Significant Other's Home	Contracts	2 hrs.	3 + 4
V. Generalization	Pt. Generates Contracts for Outside Environment	100% C.S.	Patient	Real World	Contracts	2 hrs.	5 + 6
VI. Follow-Up	Pt. Integrates Life Changes	100% C.S.	Patient	Real World	Life Impact Assessment	3 hrs.	8, 10, 14, 18
					TOTAL	15 hrs.	18 wks.

conversation, and the self-monitoring paradigm. She then approached Ms. Mapes within the home environment to complete the contract and evaluate her performance. These contracts were implemented in the home and occurred daily over a two-week period. The clinician checked the patient and significant other contracts once a week. In Phase V, the patient made and fulfilled contracts for communicative interactions in the outside environment over a two-week period. In Phase VI, the patient was seen on a systematic schedule to determine the permanence and durability of her behavioral changes and to measure the impact of these changes on her life system. Four hours of professional time were provided. She was seen first on a biweekly basis and then on a once a month basis. Her total time in treatment was fifteen hours over an eighteen week period.

Conversational speech was the focus of all speech and language treatment sessions. At first the clinician measured certain parameters of the patient's motor speech and linguistic ability, but as soon as possible the patient was trained to self-monitor and self-evaluate her speech production. The semantic content of conversations was developed so that patient problem solving was fostered. Specifically, the areas of cognitive coping in which she was experiencing difficulty were strengthened. The motor speech problems presented by this patient were essentially treated by training the patient to self-monitor and evaluate her successful speech abilities and build on those successes. The clinician focused on helping the patient overcome her coping and compliance difficulties.

Occupational Therapy

As shown in Table 11.2, the O.T. program was integrated into the speech treatment program. During the diagnostic evaluation, no basic problems in ADLs were noted in the simulation stations unless speaking was required. Further, Ms. Royer did well on cognitive tasks which required limited verbal output. However, she had withdrawn from nearly all daily activity. Therefore, it was hypothesized that she required training to regain control over her daily activities as her speech improved. Thus, during Phase III when Ms. Royer was ready to self-monitor and evaluate her newly mastered communicative success, she was enrolled in O.T. During these sessions, she transferred her new speech as she interacted with the O.T. in the CIL simulation laboratories. The total time in Phase III was four hours, which occurred during the first two weeks.

In Phase IV, when the patient transferred to nonclinical environments, the patient developed contracts in which her significant other, Ms. Mapes, was asked to help her in performing ADLs in the home.

TABLE 11.2
Occupational Therapy Treatment Plan

PHASE	STIMULUS	GOAL	EVALUATOR	LOCATION	COVARIABLES ASSESSMENT	PROFESSIONAL TIME	WEEK
I. Training Target Behavior	None Needed						
II. Independent Self-Management	None Needed						
III. Transfer to Clinical Environments	O.T. Uses Interviewing Tactics in ADLS	100% C.S.	Patient	O.T.	HIA ACA	4 hrs.	1 + 2
IV. Transfer to Non-Clinical Environments	Significant Other Accompanies Pt. in ADLS	100% C.S.	Patient	Significant Other's Home	Contracts	2 hrs.	3 + 4
V. Generalization	Pt. Engages in ADLS Alone	100% C.S.	Patient	Outside World	Contracts	2 hrs.	5 + 6
VI. Follow-Up	Speech Clinician						
					TOTAL	8 hrs.	6 Wks.

The patient was assisted by Ms. Mapes in cooking, cleaning, laundry, and engaging in general activities within the household. This occurred on a contract basis over two weeks and required two hours of professional time. In Phase V, Generalization, the patient began to engage in ADLs outside the home environment. First, the patient was accompanied by Ms. Mapes in shopping and banking excursions. By the end of this phase, the patient was able to manage all necessary ADLs by herself. Again, treatment occurred over a two week period and required two hours of professional time. Phase VI, Follow-up sessions, was conducted by the speech pathologist on a systematic schedule. The total number of professional hours devoted to O.T. was eight hours over a six week period.

Pharmacological Intervention

For treatment of her clinical depression, Ms. Royer began on Tofranil, 50 mg. p.o. daily. Over the first two weeks, her insomnia diminished and her anorexia improved. At the end of the second week, her serum imipramine level was subtherapeutic. Her Tofranil was increased to 100 mg. p.o. daily. Over the following month, her mood elevated and her fatigue disappeared. Her subsequent serum imipramine level was therapeutic. The impact of the speech treatment and occupational therapy was to accelerate the resolution of the depression.

RESULTS

Following fifteen hours of speech therapy and eight hours of O.T. delivered over an eighteen week period, the patient's mean length of utterance increased from 2.6 to 13.8 in the clinic and from 3.4 to 12.9 in the environment. Communicative success, appropriateness, and comprehension as measured on the *Adult Communicative Analysis* (ACA) increased from 68% and 40% to 100% in the clinic and environment respectively. As the treatment program progressed, the patient's speech intelligibility improved as well. Although she continued to make apraxic errors as her utterance length increased, she offered the listener additional information so that decoding the message was possible. Although transfer away from the clinic was not scheduled until Phase IV, both the patient and Ms. Mapes reported that she began to show notable improvement outside the clinic in the second week of therapy. At follow-up, she reported that she had rented her own apartment and purchased new furniture, taking great pleasure in decorating a new home. She regained complete control over her finances and reestablished her role as the church organist. She returned to her social clubs and began to entertain her friends. She reported that she felt she was able to manage her life as independently as she did prior to her stroke, stating that she "now had the world by the tail." Readministration of the coping and compliance assessment indicated that all parameters were within normal limits by the eighteenth week of her treatment.

REFERENCES

Florance, C. (1975). *Diagnostic Treatment Protocols for Apraxia of Speech*. Rehabilitation Services Administration Technical Report.

Florance, C. (1981). Methods of communication analysis used in family interaction therapy. In R. Brookshire (Ed.), *Clinical Aphasiology Conference Proceedings*. Minneapolis: BRK Publishers.

Florance, C. (1982). *The coping and compliance assessment*. NIH Technical Report.

Florance, C. (1984). *Assessment of support system*. Unpublished. Center for Independent Living Research and Training Module.

Florance, C. (1984). *Analysis of interaction dynamics*. Unpublished. Center for Independent Living Training and Research Module.

Porch, B.E. (1967). *Porch Index of Communicative Ability*. Palo Alto, CA: Consulting Psychologists Press.

Wechsler, D. (1955). *Wechsler Adult Intelligence Scale*. San Antonio, TX: Psychological Corporation.

CHAPTER 12
A Social Communication Approach to Treatment of Aphasia in an Institutional Setting
Rosemary Lubinski

> Clients living in institutional settings frequently present severe speech and language deficits. Because they are isolated from society, these individuals may be afforded few opportunities for communication. Lubinski details the use of a social communication approach with a severely aphasic woman in a nursing home. Treatment focused on maximizing the client's residual communication skills in her environment, prompting her caregivers to see her as a viable communication partner and stimulating them to become involved in the treatment process. Lubinski's report indicates a need to "rethink" the manner in which speech and language services are provided to institutionalized aphasic persons.

1. What premises underlie the use of a social communication approach in aphasia treatment? What were some of Lubinski's observations of the patient that prompted the change from traditional treatment to the social communication approach to treatment? What are the benefits of conducting treatment outside the treatment room?
2. What procedures does the author employ in drawing nursing home staff and other patients into the treatment activity? What were some of the problems in accomplishing this? Describe the author's feelings and apprehensions about using the social communication paradigm.
3. What problems are faced in documenting treatment results with Lubinski's approach? How did the author assess changes in the client and in her caregivers' reactions? What types of aphasic clients would you expect to find in a nursing home? Is the social communication approach presented by Lubinski appropriate for these clients? Why or why not?

INTRODUCTION

Increasing opportunities for aphasic clients living in nursing homes to use their limited communication skills provides a special challenge for the speech-language pathologist. These severely aphasic clients are typically chronic, elderly, and reflect cognitive, perceptual-motor, and other deficits that are compounded by the effects of aging, institutionalization, and isolation from the world. These patients are not the "model cases" for aphasia textbooks. They require treatment that is distinctively different from that offered most aphasic patients for several reasons.

Severity of Aphasia. The fact that severely aphasic patients do not respond robustly to traditional aphasia treatment is well known (Marshall, Tompkins, Rau, Philips, & Golper, 1979; Sarno & Levita, 1981; Sarno, Silverman, & Sands, 1970). These individuals, however, show a disparity between their formal test performance and their competence in functional communication situations. These disparities have been described previously (Fioldi, Cicone, & Gardner, 1983; Davis & Wilcox, 1981; Holland, 1982). A social-communication approach is intended to "tap" these residuals and enhance the patient's functional communication (Towey & Pettit, 1980; Aten, Caligiuri, & Holland, 1982). 1982).

The Environment. The impact of environment, particularly the nursing home environment, on communication has been described in some detail by Lubinski (1981a, 1981b) and Lubinski, Morrison, and Rigrodsky (1981). She suggests that the typical nursing home is a communicatively impoverished environment where the aphasic person has (a) few communication partners, (b) little reason to communicate, (c) no place to talk privately, and (d) encounters many physical and psychosocial barriers to communication. Other writers have documented these observations. Holland (1980) in collecting normative data for the *Communicative Activities of Daily Living* (CADL) found that nonaphasic institutionalized subjects performed poorer on the test than nonaphasic subjects who did not live in institutional settings. Baskey (1982) noted that nursing home aides talked less and in a more "mothering" fashion to elderly demented patients than to patients not having this diagnosis.

Incorrect Perceptions Although aphasic persons in a nursing home usually have severe speech and language deficits, their ability to function as communicators is rarely considered. Caregivers may not view them as viable communication partners and may feel awkward talking to them. Too frequently, caregivers avoid interactions with these patients and demand little from them in terms of using the skills they do have. Many caregivers view communication, other than that necessary for daily care, as a serendipitous byproduct of quality nursing and rehabilitation care. In short, the aphasic patient in the nursing home is usually talked *to* rather than talked *with*. Their needs are anticipated; opportunities to communicate and interact, other than those associated with daily care, are limited.

A SOCIAL COMMUNICATION APPROACH

Underlying Assumptions

If aphasic persons in nursing homes are to use their limited communicative residuals, they need opportunities for communication that exceed those given in treatment sessions with the speech-language pathologist. These opportunities can only be provided by persons in their environment (e.g., nurse, aide, secretary, occupational and physical therapist, and other patients). This necessitates that these persons accept the aphasic patient as a viable communication partner regardless of his or her level of functioning. Attitudes must be changed and members of the environment need to be guided to view the patient differently and to break down communication barriers. Clinicians need to determine the most efficacious way to treat these clients, while patients must be led to realize the rewards of using the residuals skills they possess in as productive a fashion as possible.

The treatment approach outlined in this chapter stems from the philosophy that in the nursing home effective treatment must constantly consider the nature of the social communicative environment as part of the therapeutic endeavor. To improve cognitive, perceptual, and linguistic skills without providing opportunities for communication is similar to asking a swimmer to practice in an empty pool. Communication skills have significance only when they have a functional context in which to be used. Speech pathologists must not assume that aphasic clients return to environments that encourage them to use their skills after treatment. Thus, if our goal is meaningful communication, the burden for improvement must be shared by the aphasic individual and members of his or her environment.

This approach to aphasia presumes that significant others in the environment will need to accept unconditionally the aphasic person as a potential partner while deliberately creating situations where communication might occur. Significant others must learn communication strategies for eliciting the best possible communication skills from the aphasic person. Further, they must realize that communication failure on the part of the aphasic must not be followed by withdrawal from that partner. The quality of interaction with the severely impaired aphasic is not measured by the quantity of verbal output or the accuracy of syntactic complexity, but by the patient's willingness to attempt to communicate even in the face of severe difficulty. The significant others in the environment must realize that *they* are the *crucial* ingredients in the communication of the severely impaired aphasic person. *They* are the sources of information and activities that produce topics and reasons for communication. *They* are the individuals who can minimize the physical barriers and increase opportunities for communication.

This case report describes the treatment of Wanda, a 78-year-old severely aphasic woman. Wanda resides in a nursing home, and it is anticipated that she will remain there the rest of her life. Treatment was intended to enhance her use of social communication in her nursing home environment. This chapter details some of the issues that need to be addressed in treating institutionalized aphasic adults, not the least of which is the need for "rethinking" the clinical procedures used in managing such individuals.

THE CASE: WANDA

Wanda suffered a left hemisphere stroke with resulting right hemiplegia and severe aphasia in August 1979, two years prior to being referred to the speech pathology consultant. Medical records obtained from the nursing home did not provide details on the extent of her lesion, but suggested she had suffered several previous milder strokes. Wanda received no speech and language therapy during a two year stay in an acute care hospital as she awaited placement in the nursing home. These two years were also devoid of other rehabilitation efforts. During this time, Wanda established a close bond with another woman who was placed in the same nursing home and became her roommate. When she was referred for a speech and language evaluation, her medical condition was stable. Her care plan specified that she needed "full assistance in all daily care," and placed particular emphasis on management of her diabetes, her incontinence, and reduction of her ankle edema. Although she received physical and occupational therapy for six months following placement in the nursing home, she had no functional use of her right side and was wheelchair bound.

Wanda's social history revealed that she was a first generation, unmarried Polish-American who grew up in an ethnically homogeneous community. She had completed the ninth grade and worked in a number of custodial and kitchen-helper positions until she retired at age 65. Her only living relatives were an elderly sister-in-law and several nieces and nephews. Except for an occasional holiday visit by her sister-in-law, she had no visitors.

Speech and Language Evaluation

I evaluated Wanda two months after her admission to the nursing home. Administration of selected portions of the *Minnesota Test for Differential Diagnosis of Aphasic* (MTDDA) (Schuell, 1965) showed her to have pervasive deficits in all language modalities. She produced no spontaneous speech during the testing situation. Those few verbal productions that I could elicit from Wanda consisted of one-word utterances that were paraphasic errors and frequently perseverative. Her speech reflected a slight Polish accent with mild apraxia of speech. Wanda did not appear to be aware of her errors and made no attempts to self-correct them. She was unable to name objects or to produce automatic speech (e.g., counting, days of the week), and performance on simple repetition tasks was markedly impaired, even when combined visual, gestural, and auditory cues were used as facilitators. Her auditory comprehension was severely impaired even for the simplest of tasks. For example, she was unable to point to objects, letters, or body parts; she had no functional reading or writing.

While Wanda reflected speech and language deficits fitting the textbook descriptions of severe or global aphasia (Collins, 1983; Helm-Estabrooks, 1984), there was a "bright spot." Her auditory comprehension in context was better than that seen in formal test performance. For example, when asked "What time is it?" she pointed to the clock on the wall, but she could not point to the picture of the clock on the first subtest of the MTDDA. Finally, she seemed to enjoy communicative interaction.

TREATMENT

I began seeing Wanda for speech and language treatment in December of 1981. She was brought to my office and we worked together on (a) improving her auditory comprehension for yes-no questions related to activities of daily living and her surroundings; (b) increasing verbal production and gestural representation of functional words and phrases; (c) improving her ability to categorize objects and concepts in her environment; and (d) reducing her perseverative responses. Although this traditionally based treatment progressed adequately, my observations of Wanda in other areas of the nursing home suggested that her communicative competence in her environment was different than what the testing and therapeutic contexts revealed.

Observations

Each day I returned with Wanda to her room after our treatment session. I usually made few remarks to Wanda's roommate. At these times

Wanda attempted to join in the conversation and, surprisingly, her unsolicited comments were often appropriate. I asked her roommate if she and Wanda talked together and she replied "Oh, you can't talk to her," suggesting that she did not consider Wanda a viable communication partner. This comment prompted me to spend more time observing Wanda in the nursing home to determine who talked with her, the frequency, the subject, and the success of these communications. I observed that Wanda was highly sociable. She smiled at everyone, waved, and often said "Hi ja." She attempted communication with staff and other patients, but their follow-up remarks were generally brief and as appropriately described by Shakepeare's Hamlet as "weary, stale, flat and unprofitable." Unfortunately, while this severely aphasic individual wanted to communicate, physical, social, and attitudinal problems in her environment precluded it.

The Environment

Wanda resided in a 200-bed nursing home in a large metropolitan city. Her care was funded by Social Security and Medicaid. Her floor housed a mixture of patients who required skilled nursing services. It contained three wings of 15 single or double occupancy rooms. All of Wanda's physical and daily care needs were met on this floor. Her double occupancy room was separated by a sliding curtain. She had few personal possessions on her side of the room, and her roommate's half of the room was equally barren of personalization. Neither woman had a television set, radio, or telephone.

Wanda was required to dress each day and to eat two meals in a communal dining room. However, she spent most of each day in a wheelchair outside her room with her roommate. Their room was the last on the corridor and they could view the length of the hallway leading toward the nurse's station. Few visitors or staff come to this end of the hall unless specifically required to do so.

The staff on Wanda's floor consisted of two registered nurses, two practical nurses, and four to six aides. During the late afternoon and evening shifts fewer staff were present. Wanda's physician visited her monthly for a required examination. Similarly, the social worker stopped by occasionally as did other staff and volunteers. Wanda had opportunities to participate in a variety of activities in adjacent sections of the nursing home, but she was dependent on staff to transport her to the activity, although her occasional incontinence discouraged participation. She attended weekly Catholic Mass and occasionally participated in group activities on her floor. At the time of her speech evaluation, the nursing supervisor summarized Wanda's behavior as "Cooperative, cheerful, with periods of confusion" and described her language as incomprehensible.

In summary, Wanda lived in an environment in which there were few opportunities for her to communicate and many barriers to using the communication skills she did have. Observation in a relaxed and natural context revealed she had some potential to communicate her thoughts and feelings, but our traditional treatment sessions did not "tap" these strengths. A different treatment approach was needed.

Changing Directions

Wanda's treatment goals took the following questions into account:

1. Was treatment facilitating Wanda's functional communication needs when she returned to her floor?
2. Did the environment contain communication partners who interacted with her and reinforced her for communicating?
3. Was her clinical communication profile commensurate with what she appeared to be able to do in social interactions within her environment?
4. Would the most successful treatment result in her being perceived as other than a severely aphasic person?

In each case the answer was no, therefore, I established the following new treatment goals for Wanda:

1. Increase Wanda's viability as a communication partner on her floor, particularly with her roommate, staff most involved with her care, and with patients with whom she often came in contact.
2. Increase her opportunities to use social communication, particularly overlearned phrases (e.g., Hi! How are you) that might "spark" an interaction with another person.
3. Increase her ability to follow changes in conversation topics during conversation.
4. Increase the number of interactions generated by staff members with Wanda.

Treatment Strategies

My first priority was to portray Wanda as a potential communication partner to the staff and other patients. Instead of seeing Wanda in my office, I conducted treatment at the end of the hall near Wanda's room or adjacent to the nurse's station where there was a steady flow of observers. I included Wanda's roommate in the treatment session so that she, Wanda, and I were involved in a communication group. I generated topics and attempted to keep discussion and conversation flowing. This activity immediately attracted the attention of patients and staff who expressed interest in our conversation.

To enable Wanda to contribute to the conversation, I elicited from her production of social phrases that she often used appropriately. For example, a treatment session might begin as follows:

Clinician: What's new ladies? How's it going?

Roommate: Same as ever.

Clinician: And you, Wanda?

Wanda: So, so. Not so good.

Clinician to Roommate: What's the matter with Wanda?

Roommate: I don't know. Ask her.

Clinician: What's wrong, Wanda? Tell me.

Wanda: Not so good. (motions to swollen leg propped up)

This discourse demonstrates Wanda's use of the perseverative response, "so, so" in an appropriate context. Furthermore, the roommate told me to elicit the information from Wanda, suggesting that she viewed Wanda as being capable of making this response.

One topic that generated a lively conversation was the subject of bachelors. With tongue in cheek, I suggested that Wanda should "keep her eyes open" for a rich bachelor around the nursing home. This statement prompted the following conversation:

Clinician: You know, Wanda, while you're sitting around here, you should keep your good eye open for a bachelor. You know the saying, it's never too late.

Wanda: A bachelor?

Clinician: Yeah you know, not married.

Wanda: For me?

Clinician: For both of us. An older one for you and a younger one for me. What do you think of that?

Wanda: Oh, you're kidding. (laughs)

Clinician: No, you've got plenty of time to sit here. Just watch who's available.

Roommate: That's all we do here. Sit.

Clinician: So, you keep a look out for us both, Wanda. Two bachelors, maybe. Maybe a father and a son.

Wanda: You rich one?

Clinician: Do I want a rich one? What other kind is there?

Wanda: I don't know. Rich one. (laughs)

Nurses' Aide: What are you all laughing about down here?

This vignette demonstrates how Wanda followed the conversation, participated by using social phrases such as "you're kidding," and "I don't know," and generated questions appropriate to the context. In addition, much laughing occurred within this interaction. The amusing topic of bachelors elicited winks and smiles from Wanda, and she apparently comprehended my use of idiomatic phrases. More important, it attracted the attention of the nurse's aide who wanted to know what was being talked about. Subsequently she was included in the conversation.

As a second priority I made a concerted effort to involve Wanda's roommate, nursing home staff, and other patients in our conversations. To accomplish this I introduced topics that had high interest for the other older patients, and then reinforced these individuals for responding to or following through on Wanda's comments. Topics included housework, cooking, gardening, World War II, the Depression, old photographs, shopping, and getting married. Ultimately, I gradually removed myself as the primary communicator in the situation.

The following sample illustrates how I encouraged Wanda to ask questions and reinforced her communication partners for participating in the interaction.

Clinician: What a day. I'm pooped out.

Wanda: Why you pooped out?

Clinician: I'm spring cleaning at home. Know what I've been doing?

Wanda: No. what?

Clinician: What have I been doing? Well, washing windows, scrubbing the floors.

Wanda: You work hard.

Resident: Yeah, that's hard work.

Clinician to Resident: What kind of things did you do during spring cleaning at home?

Resident: I always cleaned our attic every spring.

Clinician: What did you do, Wanda, during spring cleaning?

Wanda: Do?

Resident: Yeah. She asked you how you did your spring cleaning. You must have done it back then. They don't clean like that any more. No they don't.

Wanda: No, not any more. Not much.

Clinician: Your friend here asked you what you did during spring cleaning. Tell us.

Resident: I bet you were a clean one. I can tell.

Wanda: Oh, work hard. You too? What you do?
(to Resident 2)

During these conversations I encouraged Wanda to use social phrases that would be appropriate to the context. I also prompted her to ask questions that would involve her in the conversation. For example:

Clinician: Ask Mary how old her grandchildren are.

Wanda: How old your children?

Wanda quickly picked up this strategy. To avoid having it seem as if had told her what to say, I used closure phrases that would elicit an appropriate comment from Wanda but still maintain her conversational turn if it appeared she was not participating through her self-initiated words or phrases. The following example illustrates how Wanda could be drawn into the conversation through use of a closure phrase. In fact, this one capitalized on her ability to sing familiar songs.

Clinician: Well, it's looking like the holiday season around here, ladies.

Resident: Yeah, all the stuff they put up.

Clinician: I love to decorate our house at this time of year. Makes me feel in the spirit of things.

Resident: Yeah, me, too. But I don't put the things up, they do. (points to aides hanging decorations)

Clinician
(to Wanda): It's getting to look a lot like _____.

Wanda:	Christmas. Everywhere we go. (maintains melody of song)
Resident:	Even in the dining room. All over they're decorating.
Wanda:	Beautiful, everywhere, beautiful.

I also modeled other techniques for staff and patients to demonstrate Wanda's communicative competence. One of these, the use of combined gestures and verbal production, appeared to increase her comprehension and expression. For example, in the interaction about rich bachelors, I used a hand gesture to indicate money. Nursing home staff were also shown that if they took the time to introduce Wanda to the topic, even though it required several repetitions, she would become an active participant. In the following conversation about flower bouquets this participation is clearly illustrated.

Clinician:	Someone left a bouquet down by the desk. Did you notice it, Wanda?
Wanda:	A bouquet?
Clinician:	A beautiful bunch of flowers. Daisies, roses, in a lovely vase. You know, a bouquet.
Roommate:	Yeah, you have one right there on your table.
Wanda:	Them flowers.
Clinician:	That's right. You have some right behind you. Let's see what's in your vase.
Wanda:	Roses.
Clinician:	I don't know what these little white ones are.
Wanda:	I don't know; you know? (to roommate)
Roommate:	They're artificial. The ones down there are real. Real ones. You know, they smell.
Wanda:	How you know that?
Roommate:	I saw them right there. You did, too.
Wanda:	I see them?
Roommate:	We passed them going to lunch. Somebody must have brought them.
Wanda:	Oh, must be nice.

TREATMENT OUTCOMES

Wanda received social communication treatment twice weekly for 30 minute sessions for six months. I conducted treatment at lunch, during nursing home activities, in the hallway, near the nurses' station, and wherever there was a person who observed us, that person was encouraged to participate in our conversation. Treatment was terminated gradually, and I eventually stopped my direct contact with Wanda and simply "stopped by to say hello." As this reduction in treatment occurred, I reviewed the purpose of social communication treatment with the staff and the importance of their role in the initiation of conversation with Wanda. Whenever I saw a staff member interact with Wanda, I reinforced that individual for their participation with a compliment.

To document treatment outcomes, I obtained two 10-minute samples of Wanda's communicative interactions. One involved Wanda and a staff member, and the other involved Wanda, the clinician, and a student intern. I also observed Wanda sitting by the nurses' station and charted the nature and frequency of her interchanges with staff and patients. In addition, the MTDDA was readministered.

Environment Change

There were a number of observable changes in Wanda's communication. During two fifteen-minute periods of observation, Wanda initiated three and five interactions respectively with staff or residents. Although this interaction consisted of her typical "Hi ja?" or "What's new?" these social phrases prompted appropriate and interesting comments to Wanda by the staff members. Furthermore, during these 15-minute periods, two staff members and two patients initiated comments to Wanda. In these situations Wanda's responses to the staff were relevant to the topic, but contained semantic and syntactic errors.

In analyzing Wanda's taped conversations with the staff member and with the therapist and student intern, I saw that she also generated appropriate single words or short phrases (2 to 5 words), made topic shifts successfully more than 80% of the time, asked questions, and decreased the number of her verbal perseverations.

Several nursing staff staff members were asked to describe how Wanda talked. Typical replies were "Oh, Wanda, you know she talks pretty good most of the time," or "Ya, gotta keep talking to her. Then she talks better, ya know."

Unfortunately, readministration of the MTDDA revealed no changes in Wanda's auditory comprehension or verbal expression subtests. Her test performance continued to show her to be severely impaired in all communicative channels.

Although I could not specifically document it, one other change appeared to occur in the nursing home environment. The staff's involvement in the use of the social communication approach with Wanda seemed to influence the frequency with which they initiated communication with all the patients.

Clinician Changes

As the clinician, I made some changes during my six months of treatment of Wanda. At first I felt uncomfortable because I was not working in my office. I felt that others would see me as only "socializing with my patient." Once a fellow clinician confronted me with "I hear you're only talking to the patients. What's Medicare going to think about that?" I needed to remind myself that it was important for other staff to see me talk with Wanda, and that getting them involved was more important than what we could accomplish with traditional treatment. Fortunately, Wanda's response to the social communication treatment and the participation of her caregivers in this process quickly squelched my uncomfortable feelings.

Problems in Utilizing a Social Communication Approach

The social communication approach appears to require little preparation. In actuality I spent considerably more time researching ideas for topics that might be of interest to older patients, reading their files to ascertain their backgrounds and interests, and setting the stage for various communication interactions in the nursing home than I would have by bringing Wanda to my office and "drilling" her on "point to" and repetition tasks. Wanda's responses, and those of the staff indicated that it was more meaningful for Wanda to experience some communicative success, to use her residual skills, and to get staff and patients involved in communicating with her than it was to continue with traditional treatment.

Three problems emerged from my treatment of Wanda. The first was my acceptance that what I was doing constituted aphasia treatment. A second problem involved stimulating patients and staff to participate in the conversations. Although they were "curious" as to what was being talked about, most preferred to listen rather than to participate. This reluctance subsided as they perceived that I was truly interested in involving them in Wanda's treatment, and that their participation was valued. (It was important to avoid conveying the idea that they *must* talk with Wanda. This demand would have stigmatized her rather then portrayed her as a potential conversational partner.)

The third problem involved the documentation of treatment gains. I made progress notes that reflected my "day-to-day" observations and estimates of progress. Retrospectively, the collection and analysis of interactional data may have offered a better means of documenting progress in a case study of this type.

CONCLUDING REMARKS

Wanda's case reminds us that there are many roads to take in aphasia treatment. Aphasic clients are diverse in their characteristics and needs, and treatment approaches must also be similarly diverse in their creativity and application. The social-communication approach described in this chapter is only one approach that stresses the improvement of functional communication skills. As a rider must have a bicycle, a swimmer a pool, individuals with aphasia must have an environment that will consciously, meaningfully, and genuinely involve them in communicative interaction. This report underscores that need.

REFERENCES

Aten, J., Caligiuri, M., & Holland, A. (1982). The efficacy of functional communication for chronic aphasic patients. *Journal of Speech and Hearing Disorders, 47*, 93–96.

Baskey, P. (1982). *Aides' communication to the elderly patients in a nursing home.* Unpublished masters thesis. University Park, PA: Pennsylvania State University.

Collins, M. (1983). Global aphasia: Knowledge in search of understanding. *Communicative Disorders, 8*, 125–137.

Davis, A., & Wilcox, J. (1981). Incorporating parameters of natural conversation in aphasia treatment. In R. Chapey (Ed.), *Language intervention strategies in adult aphasia.* Baltimore: Williams & Wilkins.

Fioldi, N., Cicone, M., & Gardner, H. (1983). Pragmatic aspects of communication in brain damaged patients. In S. Segalowitz (Ed.), *Language functions and brain organization.* New York: Academic Press.

Helm-Estabrooks, N. (1984). Severe aphasia. In A. Holland (Ed.), *Language disorders in adults.* San Diego: College Hill Press.

Holland, A. (1980). *Communicative Abilities in Daily Living.* Austin, TX: PRO-ED.

Holland, A. (1982). Observing functional communication in aphasic adults. *Journal of Speech and Hearing Disorders, 47*, 50–56.

Lubinski, R. (1981a). Environmental language intervention. In R. Chapey (Ed.), *Language intervention strategies in adult aphasia.* Baltimore: Williams & Wilkins.

Lubinski, R. (1981b). Speech, language, and audiology programs in home health care agencies and nursing homes. In D. Beasly and G.A. Davis (Eds.), *Aging: Communication processes and disorders.* New York: Grune and Stratton.

Lubinski, R., Morrison, E., & Rigrodsky, S. (1981). Perception of spoken communication by elderly chronically ill patients in an institutional setting. *Journal of Speech and Hearing Disorders, 46*, 405–412.

Marshall, R., Tompkins, C., Rau, M., Phillips, L., & Golper, L. (1979). Speech and language services for severely aphasic patients: Some professional considerations. In R. Brookshire (Ed.), *Clinical Aphasiology Conference Proceedings*. Minneapolis: BRK Publishers.

Sarno, M.T., & Levita, E. (1981). Some observations on the nature of recovery in global aphasia after stroke. *Brain and Language, 13*, 1–12.

Sarno, M.T., Silverman, M., & Sands, E. (1970). Speech therapy and language recovery in severe aphasia. *Journal of Speech and Hearing Research, 13*, 607–623.

Schuell, H. (1965). *Minnesota Test for Differential Diagnosis of Aphasia.* Minneapolis: University of Minnesota Press.

Towey, M.P., & Pettit, J.M. (1980). Improving communication competence in global aphasia. In R. Brookshire (Ed.), *Clinical Aphasiology Conference Proceedings*. Minneapolis: BRK Publishers.

CHAPTER 13

A Cognitive Approach to the Treatment of Aphasia

Roberta Chapey

> *Chapey's contribution underscores the fact that speech is the result of thought and not vice versa. She describes a cognitively based treatment approach with a 59-year-old aphasic client who performed within normal limits on standardized tests but was frustrated by his inability to communicate with people, solve problems, and make decisions.*

1. According to Chapey, what mental operations support language? List some of the evaluative tasks that "tap" the patient's ability to perform these operations.
2. What are the consequences of ignoring the communication difficulties of patients who perform well on standardized measures such as the PICA but still complain of difficulty in communicating? What points can be made to support the provision of treatment to Chapey's patient? What arguments can be made against providing treatment?
3. Differentiate between divergent and convergent production tasks. Make a list of divergent and convergent tasks that have a functional relationship to daily living activities (e.g., making a grocery list).
4. Much of what Chapey did in treatment was conversationally oriented. What structure was provided? How were treatment results assessed?

Introduction

Normal language depends upon the efficient action and interaction of its supporting cognitive processes. Cognitive approaches to the management of adult aphasia are based on the premise that aphasic persons suffer a reduction in the efficiency of these processes (Martin, 1979). Chapey (1983, 1986) operationally defines these supporting processes in terms of five mental operations contained within the Guilford (1967) Structure of Intellect Model: cognition, memory, convergent thinking, divergent thinking, and evaluation. Cognition involves knowing, awareness, immediate discovery or rediscovery, recognition of information in various forms, and understanding. Guilford (1967) used the term *cognition* to refer to the single mental operation of recognition or understanding. Neisser (1967), however, and others use the term to refer to all of the mental processes by which sensory information is transformed, reduced, elaborated upon, recovered, and used.

Memory signifies the insertion of newly acquired information into storage. *Convergent thinking* involves the generation of logical conclusions from given information, whereas *divergent thinking* refers to the generation of logical alternatives from given information emphasizing variety, quantity and relevance of output, and a readiness to change the direction of one's responses. *Evaluative thinking* or judgment is the ability to use knowledge to make appraisals, comparisons, and to formulate evaluations in terms of known specifications. Complex behaviors such as spontaneous conversation, problem solving, and decision making involve the use of two or more of these mental operations. The specific operations involved depend upon the nature of the problem solving, decision making, or communicative tasks.

Within the Guilford model, complexity can also be viewed hierarchically in terms of those "products" needed to complete the communication. From simple to complex these products might include units, classes, relations, systems, transformations, and implications (Chapey, 1983). *Classes* include groups of items that have common properties. *Relations* are meaningful connections between items of information as might be stipulated in an analogy task. *Systems* involve organized patterns of information or interrelated and interacting parts. *Transformations* include various changes such as redefinitions, shifts, and modifications of existing information. *Implications* involve information expected, anticipated, suggested, or predicted by other information. These products of the mental operations constitute the means by which associations are derived (Guilford, 1967). Many spontaneously generated communications, or those in response to the questions, directives, or requests of others, involve one of these six products.

Within a cognitive model the language impairments of aphasic persons are seen as resulting from a thought process disorder (Wepman,

1972, 1976). Treatment is therefore directed toward stimulation of the thoughts and ideas underlying language and not toward the end products of language itself (e.g., words and sentences). Traditionally, speech and language treatment for aphasic people has concentrated on the latter. While this may be appropriate for some clients, there are others who have little difficulty using "words" but are predominantly impaired in the thought processes supporting language.

The present case report describes the use of cognitive stimulation treatment with a 68-year-old aphasic man who, despite his intact performance on conventional speech and language tests, was frustrated with his propositional language impairment and his inability to communicate meaning clearly and specifically.

THE CASE: JOHN R.

John R. was an outgoing 68-year-old, right-handed man born in New York City. He was a native English speaker and had completed high school. Prior to his retirement at age 65, he had worked 28 years as a manager of a large restaurant.

Medical History

In February of 1983 John R. was seen in the emergency room of a New York City hospital. He stated that he had incurred a prior, temporary loss of consciousness. He reported that the loss was followed by an intense headache, dizziness, feelings of numbness and weakness on his right side, and onset of moderate speech and language difficulties. A CT scan was not performed, but the clinical neurologic examination suggested that he had suffered a left hemisphere cerebrovascular accident with resulting aphasia and right-sided weakness. His brief hospital course was unremarkable, and he was discharged in early March of 1983 and referred to a home health care agency for follow up.

Social History

John's first wife had died of cancer eight years before his stroke. Two years later he married Elena who had also lost her spouse. They lived in an apartment in a middle-income neighborhood. John had three grown children from his first marriage, a 36-year-old unmarried son, a 40-year-old married daughter with three children, and a 35-year-old married daughter with two children. The daughters lived in New York and the son lived in the South. Elena also had three grown and married children (one son and two daughters) who lived in New York City.

John and Elena were attempting to cope with several stressful events at the time his stroke occurred. John's son was "rethinking" his career goals and considering a move. His oldest daughter was being treated for cancer, and Elena's son was in the hospital for spinal surgery. Two months after speech and language treatment began, John's daughter died of cancer. He was devastated by his daughter's death. He was concerned about the effect this would have on her children, their ability to care for themselves, and the fact that they did not visit him.

Speech and Language Evaluation

John was evaluated in his home in March of 1983 at approximately one-month postonset. Portions of the *Minnesota Test for Differential Diagnosis of Aphasia* (MTDDA) (Schuell, 1973) and the Verbal and Gestural subtests from the *Porch Index of Communicative Ability* (PICA) (Porch, 1971) were administered. He also received the conversational and expository speech, auditory comprehension, and oral expression subtests from the *Boston Diagnostic Aphasia Exam* (BDAE) (Goodglass & Kaplan, 1983). Nonstandardized tests given included the Gelb-Goldstein-Weigl-Scheerer *Object Sorting Test* (Goldstein & Scheerer, 1941) and several cognitive tests developed by Guilford & Hoepfner (1971).

Results. John's performance on most of the standardized speech and language measures was within normal limits or indicated only mild residual language problems. For example, he attained an Overall Verbal mean on the PICA of 14.2 and Overall Gestural mean of 14.6. These scores approximated those of normal nonaphasic persons of equivalent age. On more complex communication and problem solving tasks, John experienced considerable difficulty and frustration.

Comprehension. John's comprehension of simple messages was within normal limits, but his ability to understand more abstract material, particularly if it involved low frequency words, was impaired. He had problems understanding comparatives and passives and following complex verbal directions. He was unable to follow conversations involving more than two people and did not watch certain television programs because he could no longer understand them. While he could grasp the main ideas of a simple conversation, he had difficulty when the discussion involved multiple topics or more abstract themes were involved.

His reading comprehension was similar to that for his auditory comprehension. He did well on easy tasks such as those contained on the PICA, MTDDA, and those required for many activities of daily living (e.g., reading street signs, menus, maps, and labels). He was impaired, however, in his ability to read more complex material, in that he had difficulty in grasping the main idea, using context, and in drawing conclusions from what he read.

Memory. John's linear memory (the ability to remember items in a series) was relatively good, but higher level memory operations were impaired. For example, when he was presented with 24 pictures of common objects and asked to study and remember them, he attempted to organize the stimuli into categories and clustered some of his responses to facilitate recall. However, these organizational and clustering strategies were not as effective or as frequently employed as those seen for normal subjects (Lubinski & Chapey, 1978).

Convergent Production. Convergent production tasks require the individual to generate logical conclusions from information so as to produce the best conventional response. Most aphasia test batteries contain a high proportion of such convergent tasks (e.g., sentence completion, responsive naming, repetition). John had few difficulties with these tasks, especially those that required simple, one word responses. However, when more elaborate responses were demanded (e.g., formulating sentences, describing objects, retelling stories, giving directions, producing inferences) his impairments were noticeable.

Divergent Production. Divergent production tasks and their relevance to language production and aphasia therapy have been discussed at length by Chapey (1977a, 1977b, 1981, 1983, 1986) and others (Chapey, Rigrodsky, & Morrison, 1976, 1977). These tasks require the individual to produce a number and a variety of responses, to give multiple solutions to problems, and to generate logical possibilities applicable to given situations. Examples would be having the person state as many uses as possible for a "brick" or to tell all the ways a particular product might be improved upon (Guilford & Hoepfner, 1971). On these types of tasks John was able to produce some responses. However, his responses were not as numerous or as varied as those produced by normal subjects (Chapey, 1974). This difficulty was reflected in conversational situations by a lack of initiation and an inability to elaborate on conversational topics so as to keep a discussion going.

Evaluative Thinking. John could make concrete evaluations in terms of specific criteria such as correctness or identity. However, on the evaluative thinking tasks developed by Guilford and Hoepfner (1971), he produced substantially more errors than normal individuals (Chapey & Lubinski, 1979).

Conversational Discourse. Conversation involves the use of two or more mental abilities depending upon the nature and complexity of the interaction. John produced fairly well-structured narratives on story telling tasks and in describing procedures such as changing a tire. However, his language was reduced in quantity, complexity, and specificity by his use of simpler sentence structure, limited uses of embedded clauses, absence of dependent clauses, and lack of detail in his descriptions and explanations. In addition, word retrieval difficulties were readily apparent in conversational speech. He had problems naming objects, labeling events, coming up with specific descriptive adjectives (e.g., slimy), and specifying relationships (e.g., cousin, uncle). His spontaneous speech was often susceptible to breakdown when he could not find a specific word, and on these occasions he often "shifted" to another topic. On other occasions when he could not find a specific word he frequently assumed a passive role of nonparticipant by answering only the questions he was asked.

TREATMENT

John stated that he was "frustrated" by his speech and language impairments, particularly his problem in retrieving specific words. He was annoyed that he could no longer read as well as he had, and, in many communicative interactions, he was unable to express the exact meaning of what he wanted to say. While his difficulties might seem mild when compared to those of more severe aphasic clients, they were major obstacles to John. He was unaccepting of these difficulties and stated that he was "too embarrassed" to speak to other adults.

Speech and language treatment was scheduled for twice each week under the auspices of a home health agency. This treatment focused on two major areas: supportive counseling and stimulation of those mental processes that underlie language behavior.

Counseling

John's stroke, the deaths of his first wife and daughter from cancer, his stepson's illness, and his own son's job insecurities had lowered his self-esteem and reduced his coping and compensatory abilities. Supportive counseling focused on the family's needs, John's acceptance of his deficits, and the need for his reintegration into the community.

The social worker and I worked together in providing the counseling. Our role was to provide John and Elena information so as to encourage John to exercise more initiative and to become more self-reliant. Information designed to provide a more in-depth understanding of death and dying (Kubler-Ross, 1969) and to develop an increasing awareness of the stages of psychosocial development during adulthood and old age (Knox, 1981) was provided. John and Elena were encouraged to explore "why bad things happen to good people" (Kushner, 1981). They were asked to revise their old aspirations and to set new goals, explore the benefits of retirement, count their blessings, and reintegrate themselves into society's mainstream.

John was encouraged to abandon his dependent communicative status, to become more realistic in his expectations, and to accept greater responsibility for participation in communicative interactions. In this vein, it was helpful to examine communicative situations with high potential for failure in terms of a risk-reward ratio. Similarly, the degree to which negative evaluations of others affected John's communication was discussed, and John was provided strategies for dealing with this issue.

Cognitive Treatment

The essential aim of treatment was to improve the mental processes (cognition, memory, convergent, divergent, and evaluations) underlying language either in isolation or in various combinations. For John, treatment focused on conversations and interactions within which he was required to solve problems, make decisions, plan, and think abstractly.

In carrying out this treatment plan, a certain amount of structure was necessary. For example, the turn-taking rules of PACE as discussed by Davis and Wilcox (1981) were applied to conversational situations. These involve four principles: (a) exchanging of new information between client and patient, (b) free choice of communicative channels to convey new information, (c) equal participation by clinician and patient as senders and receivers of messages, and (d) feedback from the clinician in response to the patient's success in conveying a message. In addition, as suggested by Wepman (1972, 1976), treatment was designed to prompt John to maintain continuity of content during conversations and to embellish his ideas about the topic being discussed.

Communicative success, maintaining topic relatedness, elaboration of content, and assuming the role of speaker-initiator in conversation rather than lexical and syntactic accuracy were reinforced verbally. Specific exercises involved having John formulate solutions to the problems posed in the "Dear Abby" column in the newspaper or to Dr. Tony Grant's or Dr. David Viscott's radio programs (call-in psychologists).

At times I created a problem-solving situation for John. For example, he was asked to provide a solution to the following:

> Ted was standing in line in a grocery store. From out of nowhere, a young boy appeared, pushed Ted out of line, and took his place in line. What would you do if you were Ted?

Other examples included decision-making tasks (e.g., listing considerations in buying a house) and role playing (e.g., viewing a situation through the eyes of someone else). These were highly stimulating to John. He was also encouraged to discuss the pros and cons of ideas for global problems such as controlling inflation or personal preferences like living in an apartment.

I encouraged John to resume reading the newspaper. Initially, I asked him to scan the headlines and to speculate about the content of the article. Then I had him read the first paragraph, summarize the material, and state if the headlines predicted the content of the story. Eventually, he was given the responsibility of keeping me up to date on current events by reading and summarizing two articles that would be of interest to me. Finally, he was asked to justify these selections.

To assist John in combatting his word-retrieval difficulties in conversation, I taught him to utilize a variety of self-cueing strategies. These strategies involved the use of delays, semantic associations, phonetic associations, descriptions, asking questions, and tapping out the number of syllables in the desired word. In addition, I provided John a number of workbooks within which he carried out homework assignments that I checked at the beginning of each treatment session (Brubaker, 1983; Holloran & Bressler, 1983: Lazzari & Peters, 1980; Kilpatrick, 1979: Morganstein & Smith, 1982; Zachman, Jorgensen, Barrett, Huisingh, & Sneeden, 1982). Other materials were also employed in homework assignments and in treatment. These included cookbooks, books on sports and hobbies, newspapers, and various magazines.

Treatment also focused upon the stimulation of specific cognitive operations. During some sessions I gave John practice in recognizing individual words and word classes, either directly or from a description of their action or function. Other related tasks included arranging a series of colors in terms of brightness, ordering a set of objects by size, and categorizing objects and words. For example, I had him eliminate words that did not belong in a particular category series (e.g., cheese: muenster, swiss, cheddar, vanilla). Other tasks included rearranging scrambled words to make a meaningful sentence, recognizing problems inherent in particular situations, and understanding how the same sentence or statement might be interpreted differently (e.g., He lost his shirt).

As treatment progressed I increased the length and complexity of task stimuli. For example, I encouraged John to analyze and to order the steps he would go through in carrying out a certain operation (e.g., making soup, changing a flat tire, getting to a ball game). It was particularly helpful to have him explain how comprehension of a sentence was based on the identification of specific types of relationships (e.g., part-whole, familial, spatial, cause-effect), to identify main ideas of a discussion, and to follow topic changes in conversations.

To improve his reading comprehension I had John read paragraphs of high-interest material. I reinforced him verbally for using the context to comprehend the material, getting the main idea, detecting the sequence of events, and drawing conclusions. When he misinterpreted what he had read, I pointed out his errors and asked him to reread the paragraph and to correct the response. He was then asked to explain why he had made the error. I also assigned him reading material as homework. Particularly useful in this regard were the Barnell Loft, Ltd. (Boning, 1973) series of workbooks for which I gave John the answer key. This practice allowed him to complete independent work assignments at home and to check his work and filled a need to be doing something "on his own."

Memory. I encouraged John to try to recall and use more abstract, lower frequency words and to use organizational strategies to facilitate memory. For example, I might talk about a trip I had taken and the different types of food I had eaten. I would then ask John to try to recall what Italian dishes, French dishes, and American dishes had been eaten on my trip. This procedure was used to teach him to group ideas by category or to chunk information into meaningful units.

Convergent Production. Several convergent production tasks were used in my treatment of John. Initially, I employed simple tasks such as labeling objects, events, relationships, defining (words, relationships), describing functions, categorizing (fruits, vegetables, clothing articles), and giving synonyms, antonyms, homonyms, and rhyme words. Subsequently, I had John supply attributes of various objects (e.g., a brick, a piece of glass, an iron bar), answer questions about everyday living situations (How do you visit your doctor?), sequence steps in achieving an end product (e.g., making a pot of coffee), retell stories in terms of their literal details (who, when, what, where, how), and to draw conclusions and make inferences on the basis of the content of the story. Finally, he was asked to respond to more abstract questions such as "What is Communism?" and to solve math problems.

Divergent Production. Divergent semantic thinking exercise involved tasks such as naming all the objects he could think of that could be eaten, washed, or folded, suggesting as many things as he could that were fast, slow, or ran on gasoline, and supplying as many uses as possible for various objects (e.g., tin can, paper clip, key). I further stimulated divergent production by having John provide as many possible problems as he could for particular situations (e.g., eating a meal in a restaurant) and stipulating potential consequences for unusual situations (e.g., What might happen if clouds had strings attached that hung down to earth?).

Divergent tasks promote the generation of solutions for solving problems and encourage flexibility of thinking rather than rigidity.

Accordingly, I had John arrive at multiple solutions for handling everyday problems such as running out of gas, shopping for clothes, and lowering the crime rate. Other useful endeavors included providing ways to improve products (e.g., airplane, breadboard) and giving ways in which various objects were alike or different. I also assigned him practical tasks in which he had to detail steps of a plan, such as going on a weekend trip to the mountains with four friends, or how a particular set of clothes might be described by a six-year-old boy, a football player, a teenager, a husband, and a fashion designer.

To promote further divergent thinking within conversations, I encouraged John to think of different ways to initiate conversations, different methods of maintaining conversational flow (e.g., elaboration, verification), and how to repair conversational breakdowns (e.g., revising, asking for repeats). Finally, we discussed the social conventions followed by communicative partners in conversations (e.g., turn taking).

Evaluative Thinking. I provided John examples of situations (real and contrived) in which I had him make a judgment as to what he would do in terms of criteria such as social acceptability, safety, utility, and so forth. For example, in determining the best solution to spilling liquid on the floor, I asked "If you spill something on the floor, the best thing is to (a) let it dry, (b) wipe it up, (c) put a rug over it, or (d) scrape it up on a plate and eat it." In another task labeled "taking the first step" I asked, "If you discover a leak under your sink, what is the first thing you do? (a) call a plumber, (b) get a bucket, (c) get a pair of pliers, or (d) make sure the water is off." In another task I had him rank the cost of items from least to most expensive (e.g., house, Rolls Royce, tickets to the theater, medical school).

I found that several other activities were useful in improving John's ability to make judgments and evaluations. These activities included giving words that best fit particular situations and choosing the best two reasons (from a series of five) a particular plan might be faulty. Further, I gave him practice in identifying implications inherent in verbal absurdities and humor (e.g., "What kind of bow is impossible to tie, a ribbon or a rainbow?"). I encouraged him to evaluate the intent of specific messages, the coherency of conversations, and what should or should not be said in certain contexts, with different people, and when certain consequences were apparent.

RESULTS

Eventually, our counseling efforts and the cognitive treatment assisted John in becoming an assertive communicator. He began to initiate communication more often, and he started to venture into his neighborhood again to talk with friends and to attend the monthly meetings of the Retired Business and Professional Association (RBPA), an organization for which he had been vice president before his stroke. Ultimately, John and Elena began to go on weekend outings with RBPA members. Although John continued to "feel bad" about his physical and communicative limitations, he gradually developed a positive attitude about his ability to contribute to a conversation and to realize that it was better to risk the possibility of communicative failure than not to communicate at all.

Assessing the efficacy of cognitive treatment with a high level aphasic patient like John was difficult because there are no currently available standardized tests for this purpose. There were, however, several areas where the results of speech and language treatment were clearly evident. First, John now initiated more communication with his wife and others. Before treatment, he was a high level performer on typical standardized test batteries such as the PICA, BDAE, and MTDDA, but he was not a communicator. He avoided conversations, was embarrassed by his deficits, and frustrated with his inabilities to retrieve specific words and to express himself explicitly. Treatment improved his word retrieval skills; moreover, as this occurred, his spontaneous speech became more specific and detailed and contained a greater number of elaborations. He could, for example, provide more detail when telling the clinician how to cook manicotti, make a pay phone call, or brew a cup of espresso. Ultimately, his descriptions included more low-frequency words. John's participation in combatting his word-retrieval difficulties was also apparent. Not only did he become proficient in using self-initiated strategies to elicit a target word (e.g., delay, semantic association, Marshall, 1976), but he began to keep a list of words that were difficult to retrieve, spent hours repeating them alone, and immediately rehearsed these words for the clinician when she arrived for the treatment session.

John's use of memory strategies also improved. This result was clearly seen by increased use of clustering of items in both study time and recall. Review of homework assignments, most noticeably the reading tasks, revealed fewer and fewer errors as treatment continued. Further, his ability to locate the main idea, to use context to comprehend what he read, and to make inferences and draw conclusions improved. He read little for pleasure when treatment began, but by the end of treatment he was reading avidly material appropriate to his level of performance.

Perhaps the most appropriate summary of the effect of speech and language treatment for John is summarized by a letter from his son to the clinician following termination of treatment.

Dear Dr. Chapey,

When my father suffered a stroke and was left with a speech impairment, it was a difficult thing for him, and for the people that love him. He was always very glib, vocal and articulate with a wonderful vocabulary. I remember as a young boy, he and I would spend about an hour every Sunday playing a 'dictionary game,' challenging each other about the meaning of words. It was always fun for both of us, and now it is a cherished memory of mine. (He won most of the time!)

Language, words and speech are very important. My father always enjoyed them! The realization of their impairment took a heavy toll on him psychologically.

I have seen his improvement in his speech which has lead to an improvement in his health and mental attitude. I am very proud of Dad's inner strength and courage when faced with the tasks of rebuilding his speech. I am also very happy that you were such an important part in that difficult process. Thank you for bringing your expertise, professionalism and most important of all, your human concern, and from what Dad says, genuine interest in him and his progress. I am sure that you helped him draw on his own energies to repair and strengthen his speech. I admire you, thank you and pray that God will bless you in your important work.

REFERENCES

Boning, R. (1973). *Specific skill series.* Baldwin. NY: Barnell Loft.

Brubaker, S. (1983). *Workbook for reasoninq skills. Exercises for cognitive facilitation.* Detroit: Wayne State University Press.

Chapey, R. (1974). *Divergent semantic behavior in aphasia.* Doctoral dissertation. New York: Columbia University.

Chapey, R. (1977a). A divergent semantic model of intervention in adult aphasia. In R. Brookshire (Ed.), *Clinical Aphasiology Proceedings of the Conference.* Minneapolis: BRK Publishers.

Chapey, R. (1977b). The relationship between divergent and convergent semantic behavior in adult aphasia. *Archives of Phvsical Medicine Rehabilitation, 58,* 357–362.

Chapey, R. (1981). Divergent semantic intervention. In R. Chapey (Ed.), *Language intervention strategies in adult aphasia.* Baltimore: Williams & Wilkins.

Chapey, R., (1983). Language based cognitive abilities in adult aphasia: Rationale for intervention. *Journal of Communication Disorders, 16,* 405–424.

Chapey, R. (1986). Cognitive intervention: Stimulation of cognition, memory, convergent thinking, divergent thinking and evaluative thinking. In R. Chapey (Ed.), *Language intervention strategies in adult aphasia* (2nd ed.). Baltimore: Williams & Wilkins.

Chapey, R., & Lubinski, R. (1979). Semantic judgment ability in adult aphasia. *Cortex, 15,* 247–255.

Chapey, R., Rigrodsky, S., & Morrison, E. (1976). The measurement of divergent semantic behavior in aphasia. *Journal of Speech and Hearing Research, 19,* 664–677.

Chapey, R., Rigrodsky, S., & Morrison, E. (1977). Aphasia: A divergent semantic interpretation. *Journal of Speech and Hearing Disorders, 42,* 287–295.

Davis, G.A., & Wilcox, M.J. (1981). Incorporating parameters of natural conversation in aphasia treatment. In R. Chapey (Ed.), *Lanquage intervention strategies in adult aphasia*. Baltimore: Williams & Wilkins.

Goodglass. H., & Kaplan, E. (1983). *The assessment of aphasia and related disorders*. Philadelphia: Lea and Febiger.

Goldstein, K., & Scheerer. M. (1941). Abstract and concrete behavior an experimental study with special tests. *Psychological Monoqraphs, 53*, 2.

Guilford, J.P. (1967). *The nature of human intelligence.* New York: McGraw Hill.

Guilford, J.M., & Hoepfner, R. (1971). *The analysis of intelligence*. New York: McGraw Hill.

Holloran, S., & Bressler, E. (1983). *Cognitive reorganization: A stimulus handbook*. Tigard, OR: C.C. Publications.

Kilpatrick. K. (1979). *Therapy guide for the adult with language disorders.* (Vol. II). Akron, OH: Visiting Nurse Service.

Knox, A. (1981). Adult development. In D. Beasley and G.A. Davis (Eds.), *Aging: Communication processes and disorders.* New York: Grune and Stratton.

Kubler-Ross, E. K. (1969). *On death and dying.* New York: Macmillan.

Kushner, H. (1981). *When bad things happen to good people.* New York: Schocken Books.

Lazzari, A., & Peters, P. (1980). *Handbook of exercises for language processing.* Moline, IL: Linguisystems.

Lubinski, R., & Chapey, R. (1978). Constructive recall strategies in adult aphasia. In R. Brookshire (Ed.), *Clinical Aphasiology Conference Proceedings.* Minneapolis: BRK Publishers.

Marshall, R. (1976). Word retrieval behavior of aphasic adults. *Journal of Speech and Hearing Disorders, 41*, 444–451.

Martin, A.D. (1979). Levels of reference for aphasia therapy. In R. Brookshire (Ed.), *Clinical Aphasiology Conference Proceedings*. Minneapolis: BRK Publishers.

Morganstein, S., & Smith, M. (1982). *Thematic language stimulation.* Tucson: Communication Skill Builders.

Neisser, U. (1967). *Cognitive psychology.* New York: Appleton Century Crofts.

Porch, B. (1971). *The Porch Index of Communicative Ability.* Palo Alto: Consulting Psychologists Press.

Schuell, H. (revised by J.W. Sefer). (1973). *Differential diagnosis of aphasia with the Minnesota test*. Minneapolis: University of Minnesota Press.

Wepman, J. (1972). Aphasia therapy: A new look. *Journal of Speech and Hearing Disorders, 37*, 203–214.

Wepman, J. (1976). Aphasia: Language without thought or thought without language. *ASHA, 18*, 131–136.

Zachman, L., Jorgensen, C., Barrett, M., Huisingh, R., & Sneeden, M. (1982). Manual of exercises for expressive reasoning. Moline, IL: Linguisystems.

CHAPTER 14
A Case for Flexibility
Robert C. Marshall

> Marshall's case highlights the multiple problems that confront the clinical aphasiologist in addition to the patient's basic speech and language deficits. The author describes two different treatment courses and their outcome for a client who suffered two strokes. The incorporation of relevant patient and family concerns and the use of "serious" language in the therapeutic arena stimulated language recovery in the client. To deal with such issues effectively demands flexibility on the part of both the clinician and the patient.

1. Why wasn't the client referred for a speech and language evaluation following his first stroke? What are the positive and negative ramifications of this lack of referral? How did Marshall deal with the friction surrounding communication between the patient and his family following the first stroke?
2. Describe the procedures used by Marshall to assist his client in compensating for his auditory comprehension and word retrieval deficits. How did the author distinguish between word retrieval and word production difficulties? Why were writing and reading assigned lower priorities in treatment than speaking and listening?
3. When the patient suffered his second stroke what indicators were there that predicted he might recover from this insult? What major alterations in treatment content and focus were made following the second stroke? Why? How do these compare with the type of treatment provided after his first stroke?

BACKGROUND INFORMATION

Mack was a 51-year-old, right-handed man who suffered a left-hemisphere thromboembolic cerebrovascular accident (CVA) with resulting aphasia and right-sided weakness in June of 1973. He was a native speaker of English and had a high school education. When he suffered his stroke, he was working as a medical technician. Previous to this he had served 23 years in the Navy as a pharmacist's mate. At that time he and his wife had been married 22 years. They have six children, four of whom were still at home.

THE CASE: MACK

Medical History. On June 17, 1973, Mack was admitted to the Veterans Administration Medical Center, Portland, Oregon (VAMC) complaining of dizziness, right-sided weakness, and sensory loss of two and one half weeks duration. He reported that he had incurred similar but transitory neurologic deficits over the past two years. Neurologic examination indicated a normal mental status with intact cranial nerves. Motor strength on the right was moderately diminished, particularly in the upper extremity. Electroencephalographic (EEG) results were normal, but a brain scan revealed an area of increased isotope uptake in the left temporal-parietal area suggestive of recent infarction. Bilateral carotid angiography was performed. The right carotid injection indicated a cross-flow to the middle and anterior cerebral arteries on the left; the left injection revealed a complete occlusion of the left internal carotid at its origin with some collateral filling from the internal maxillary artery. He was considered a candidate for carotid surgery, but a decision regarding this procedure was postponed for six months pending further recovery. Mack was discharged from the hospital on July 20, 1973 and advised that he could return to work. His hospital course was described by his attending physician as "stable." While aphasia was mentioned in the medical chart, Mack was not referred to speech-language pathology.

Six months later (December 1973) Mack was readmitted to the VAMC. He had developed a cardiac arrhythmia and hypertension that was felt to be associated with job stress. His cardiac difficulties rapidly resolved and medications were prescribed for the hypertension. A consultation was also sent to speech-language pathology.

SPEECH AND LANGUAGE EVALUATION

Mack's presenting complaint was the inability to perform his job satisfactorily. His working day involved interacting with people in a variety of situations: administering medications, making out forms, filling prescriptions, and talking on the phone. He reported that he had difficulty understanding what was said to him, particularly in noisy situations or when several people were talking simultaneously. He was upset that he could no longer read or write well enough to keep records and fill prescriptions. He became angry when he could not recall words that he knew. He avoided communication by staying away from the job or by retreating to his office. Mack was also frustrated with his communication breakdowns at home; he felt his family was "against him" and attributed his hypertension to home and job stress. He was also fearful that he might have another stroke.

In conversation, Mack was sociable, gregarious, and displayed a keen sense of humor. He nodded his head knowingly, frequently saying things like "uh-huh" and "right," seeming to understand all that was said to him. If he had problems retrieving a word, he would pause, appear to think, and say "Let's see, what the heck is that?" Then he would turn to someone in the room, often his wife, who would supply the missing word for him.

Testing. Mack was evaluated during December of 1973. Tests included the *Porch Index of Communicative Ability* (PICA) (Porch, 1967); the *Minnesota Test for Differential Diagnosis of Aphasia* (MTDDA) (Schuell, 1972); the *Boston Diagnostic Aphasia Examination* (BDAE) (Goodglass & Kaplan, 1972); the *Peabody Picture Vocabulary Test* (PPVT) (Dunn, 1965); and the *Token Test* (DeRenzi & Vignolo, 1962).

Severity and Type of Aphasia. At six months postonset Mack exhibited moderately severe aphasia affecting all language modalities. Overall performance on the PICA placed him at the 49th percentile in a large random sample of left-hemisphere damaged adults. PICA subtest means indicated that his verbal-expressive and auditory comprehension abilities were higher than his written expression and his reading abilities. Percentage of correct responses on the sections of the MTDDA were auditory comprehension (88%); visual-reading (72%); speech and language (83%); and writing (46%). He received an overall severity rating of "3" on the five point BDAE severity rating scale.

Mack's expository speech performance and auditory comprehension scores for the BDAE did not categorize him as a "classical aphasia type" (Broca's, Wernicke's, Conduction, Anomic). Spontaneous speech was sometimes fluent, but on an equal number of occasions it was halting and laborious. The latter was associated with articulatory errors, word-finding problems, and difficulties in sentence formulation. A transcription of his description of the "Cookie Theft" picture from the BDAE provides a good example of his conversational speaking ability.

"She – sh she, that's a boy there and he is almost ready to fall on his ass. And the – uh – mother – her sink is over – is fl – flowing overflowing. Okay? And the – uh – and it looks like it's – uh – windy outside. Cause the – uh – billows are back and forth. And it looks like that she isn't a very good housekeeper. And he's – that little kid is ha-haing to him over the cookies in the cookie jar. But he's falling on his ass in three seconds."

Retention and Comprehension Deficits. Brookshire (1974) points out that clients with retention deficits have increasing difficulty comprehending as messages get longer. Mack retained single words and short phrases, but not longer sentences. He could follow one-stage but not two-stage commands consistently. His performance on Parts I–IV of the *Token Test*, shown in Table 14.1, reflected a retention problem. Not only did he show a decrease in performance as commands increased in length, but he tended to respond accurately to the first command and miss the second at each level of the test. Retention-based errors were also noted on repetition tasks and in his responses to yes-no and information questions. For example, his reply to the question "Can you name the first and second presidents of the United States?" was "I know you want something about a president, but I don't remember what."

Similar retention difficulties were seen in reading as well. He read single words and short sentences with little difficulty, but made errors on the paragraph comprehension subtests of the MTDDA and BDAE. Whether reading orally or silently, he tended to forget the initial por-

TABLE 14.1
Percentage of Correct Responses on the Token Test

PART	PERCENTAGE	EXAMPLE COMMAND
Part I	100%	Touch the red circle.
Part II	90%	Touch the small green square.
Part III	70%	Touch the blue square and the yellow circle.
Part IV	40%	Touch the small green circle and the large red square.
Part V	36%	Put the white circle on top of the blue square.

tions of a passage by the time he had reached the end, and it was necessary for him to read material several times before responding.

Message length was more of a deterrent to Mack's comprehension success than semantic or syntactic complexity. He had a surprisingly well preserved single word receptive vocabulary. He identified 135 of 150 items on the PPVT correctly, and in conversation he recognized many uncommon words. Similarly, he could respond accurately to short, meaningful, syntactically complex units (e.g., "Neither the boy nor the girl is jumping") and if provided a situational context, both auditory and reading comprehension were substantially enhanced. He did well answering yes-no questions about paragraphs read to him from the MTDDA and BDAE. He performed similarly after reading paragraphs to himself. When he knew the topic (e.g., golf, finances, work) of conversation, his comprehension was quite functional. Abstract commands or questions such as occur on Part V of the *Token Test* and on some of the complex ideational tests of the BDAE (e.g., "Is one pound of flour heavier than two?") were, however, more difficult for him.

Apraxia of Speech. Mack demonstrated a mild apraxia of speech as defined by Darley (1982). This was noticeable when he was asked to repeat multisyllabic words such as "torpedo" and "catastrophe" and in conversation by false starts, revisions, and articulatory groping. When verbal expressive problems were due to the apraxia, he often corrected himself. This self-correction behavior contrasted with his behavior when the problem was difficulty retrieving the word. Mack also could produce misarticulated words and phrases after they were modeled by the clinician. In general, however, he dealt poorly with his apractic "bobbles," becoming upset when these errors interfered with completion of a communicative utterance.

Severe Dysgraphia. Mack's most severe language deficits were seen in writing. Other than the ability to sign a check, a task he had practiced at length, he had no functional writing.

Word-Retrieval Difficulties. Severe word-finding difficulties were evident in conversation and on confrontation-naming tasks. Mack usually evidenced some semantic knowledge of the word he was attempting to retrieve. For example, when trying to say the word chiropractor, he said "He's not an MD but a whatchamacallit." Sometimes this information functioned as a self-cue to evoke the desired word. His attempt to say "Washington" resulted in "My friend lives in — let's see — California, Oregon, one more — Washington."

Compensatory Behaviors. Mack had adopted some communicative strategies in the hiatus between onset of aphasia and initial evaluation. One strategy was to pretend that he understood all that was said to him. While he often comprehended the "gist" of the message, he did not retain instructions, directions, or sequences longer than a few items. He stated that he did not like to ask people to repeat because he felt it made him look like a "dummy."

Mack also relied on his wife to provide missing words for him. Unfortunately, his wife was relatively unskilled at filling in the blanks. If she failed or took too long, both she and Mack became agitated. A typical example was the interaction following the question, "Where did you enlist in the Navy?"

Client: "Let's see, it was back in" (looks at wife)

Wife: "Norfork, Virginia?" (uttered with hope)

Client: "No!" (with some agitation)

Wife: "Was it San Francisco?" (uttered with even more hope)

Client: "Oh, hell no. You know, one more down." (with more agitation)

Wife: "Oh you mean San Diego?" (with relief)

Patient: "Christ sakes, yes!" (with vengeance)

By the end of this interaction, both Mack and his wife were glaring at one another.

Finally, Mack was unduly intolerant of his speech and language errors. He expected perfection, and when he could not pronounce or recall a desired word, he lost his temper. He admitted that he had "faked" his way through communication situations so he could get out of the hospital and return to work. He stated that since he had worked in a medical setting most of his life, it was easy to "pull the wool over the eyes" (his words) of his physicians.

Family Dynamics. In his home Mack had been a charming, benevolent dictator who made the money and the decisions. He was a competitor who excelled at most of what he attempted. His premorbid description of himself was that of "the life of the party." Aphasia seriously damaged his self-concept and set into motion fears for the future in terms of finances and dependence. His years in the military had been spent interacting with men and now he was surrounded by five women. When he attempted to maintain control of them with his damaged circuitry, he was not effective, and they rebelled. This upset him and he intensified his efforts. The family retaliated by questioning him, correcting his speech, and occasionally laughing at his mistakes.

TREATMENT

Mack was scheduled for outpatient speech and language treatment twice weekly. Treatment focused on six areas: (a) supportive counseling, (b) functionalizing compensatory behaviors, (c) heightening auditory comprehension, (d) minimizing apraxic struggle, (e) establishing functional writing, and (f) improving word-retrieval skills.

Supportive Counseling

The immediate aims of counseling were to reduce communicative tensions within the home. One of the ways this was done was by having the client's oldest daughter obtain a driver's license and drive him to and from treatment. She was happy to do this, and the three to four hours spent getting to and from treatment provided a needed break for the wife. The family was told that it was normal to be uncomfortable in this new situation where Mack was now with them 24 hours per day and some adjustments would need to be made. They were advised to make sure they spent time away from him and that he had some time to spend by himself.

The nature of Mack's word retrieval and comprehension deficits was explained to the family. They wanted to know how much to help Mack talk, and if he could be harmed by the frustration and stress that sometimes resulted when he had difficulty talking for himself. They were told that when Mack's communications conveyed the intended message to be accepting and not to concern themselves with articulatory accuracy, speed, and grammatical correctness. They were also advised to give him more time (within reason) to express himself and to ignore his tempests if he could not recall a specific word. While it was acceptable to provide some of the missing words if it facilitated communication, it was stressed that they not anticipate what Mack was going to say, or speak for him.

Specifically, the family was asked not to have Mack repeat, name things, or to make fun of his errors. A final issue centered on their reluctance to say no to him. Lezak (1983) has suggested that this is sometimes a problem for the healthy members in the family, since they fear that it might upset the patient and cause him to have another stroke. In Mack's presence, the family was counseled that no one, regardless of their impairment, has the right to act as a tyrant, and that it was perfectly acceptable to stand up for one's rights.

Functionalizing Compensatory Behaviors

On those occasions when Mack pretended to understand what was said, he was confronted with questions such as "Will you tell me what I said?" or "Are you sure you have that?" This attitude encouraged him to ask for repetitions. Because Mack was concerned that this would look foolish, he was advised to be more "sophisticated" in these endeavors and to say assertively "Would you repeat that so I can get all of it?" instead of "Huh?" or "What?" Another helpful technique was to have him paraphrase the message and request verification from his conversational partner. For example, if he was asked to come for treatment on Wednesday at 1:30, he would say "Wednesday, 1:30, right?" Mack made these adjustments easily since they had an immediate payoff for him.

As mentioned earlier, the family was asked not to react to Mack's temper outbursts. When he became frustrated with a word-finding problem in treatment, he was advised to stop talking and then to provide whatever semantic information he could about the word. Ordinarily, this was adequate for the clinician to guess the word. This technique also helped Mack realize that the word was not totally lost and this helped reduce his frustration. Another helpful procedure was the playing back of tape-recorded vignettes of his outbursts. This allowed him to recognize the inappropriateness of his behavior and facilitated his using more productive efforts to combat word-retrieval difficulties later in treatment.

Refocusing. Mack's expectations of himself were extremely high. To bring these into line with his existing residuals, a technique I have termed "refocusing" was applied. Refocusing involves altering the client's attitudinal set to help him concentrate on behaviors and attributes that contribute positively to functional communication in lieu of dwelling on what he cannot do because of the stroke. I began by explaining to the patient that immediately before his insult he was functioning at his highest level (100% of ability), and that just after the insult he probably hit his lowest point (0%). Then I asked him to place himself on the continuum of recovery where he thought he was presently. Mack put himself at the 50% level. He was then asked to select a spot on the continuum where he expected his progress to end, and where he would be satisfied. The only limitation was that he was not allowed to pick 100%, because he had experienced a stroke and would never be "exactly" the same person again. Mack selected 90% as his target.

This simple exercise helped Mack see how far he had to progress to achieve his goal instead of dwelling on how far he had to go to be "normal" again. This change in perspective helps clients accept reinforcement for positive communication efforts and for using compensatory strategies. Moreover, it frees them to concentrate on strengths instead of weaknesses, successes instead of failures, and the present instead of the past. When Mack began to see the positive aspects of his communication, the situation changed. He adopted an attitude of hope and gave himself credit for doing well within the limits of his neurologic residuals.

Heightening Auditory Comprehension

Mack's primary difficulties in auditory processing resulted from a reduced retention span. In part, this problem was due to a lack of attentiveness to incoming stimuli and difficulty in switching roles from speaker to listener in conversational interactions. Alerting phrases such as "Ready now" and "Listen to me" were used to prepare him for questions and commands. To facilitate his making the change from speaker to listener, statements like "Let me say something" or "I'd like to comment on that" were used. These let Mack know that it was time to stop talking and start listening.

Brief pauses of a few seconds duration, inserted at syntactical boundaries or between sentences, were also useful in enhancing retention. As suggested by Liles and Brookshire (1975), Mack retained more information when message units were given to him in meaningful "chunks." Putting a brief pause at the boundary of a two-stage command such as "Touch your right ear, and then your left knee" increased the likelihood that he would retain the command long enough to respond correctly.

Repetition tasks were also used to increase verbal retention span. This had the added advantage of helping Mack reduce his apraxic errors. Usually, he worked so hard to remember the message, he tended not to become involved in articulatory struggles. Treatment began with short phrases such as "cup of coffee" and progressed to longer units such as "a cup of black coffee" and "a cup of hot black coffee." Sequential pointing tasks were also helpful in increasing retention. A set of four to eight pictures was placed in front of Mack. He would be asked to point to two items, then three items, and so forth. In the beginning, he was only required to select the correct items. Subsequently, he was required to point to items in their sequence of presentation.

Since Mack usually comprehended messages in context, he was less than excited about working on comprehension in drill type tasks. Therefore, direct work to improve comprehension comprised but a small portion of treatment time. Most of the efforts to heighten comprehension were incorporated into tasks designed to improve expressive language skills.

Minimizing Apraxic Struggle

Oral reading and sentence repetition tasks were utilized to increase Mack's flow of speech, articulatory accuracy, and speech rate. Treatment began with short, meaningful, phonetically simple sentences such as "I want a Bud" or "Have a cold Oly" and progressed to units that were longer and more complex such as "I'll have two bottles of Budweiser and one of Olympia." Stimuli selected for these apraxic drills were designed to be relevant to his daily activities. Generally, a list of sentences was introduced in the clinic. Mack read each sentence. If he did not produce an accurate, acceptable response, the sentence was modeled and he was asked to try again. If he could still not produce an acceptable response, the item was dropped from the list. Mack was then given the list to practice at home, and the material was reviewed at the beginning of the subsequent treatment session. This easy introductory material helped begin each treatment session on a positive note, and took only a few minutes. Shortly, Mack's speech flow and articulatory accuracy improved to a point where apraxia was not a major problem. He also developed the ability to correct his misarticulations without becoming agitated.

Establishing Functional Writing

Some short-term but unsuccessful efforts were made to improve Mack's writing. While he regained the ability to write a few single words, this was done with great effort. He could sign checks and was given some practice in writing his address and the names of his family. Writing per se, however, was assigned a low priority as a treatment goal, and more emphasis was placed on verbal communication. Mack was also provided some practice in writing single letters in the hope that he might be able to use first letters of words as "cues" to prompt successful word retrieval.

Improving Word-Retrieval Skills

Much of treatment was devoted to improving word-retrieval abilities. In the initial stages of treatment this involved the use of cueing strategies and confrontation naming tasks. Typical techniques involved the use of the first letter or syllable, description, or sentence completion. Examples of these cues for the item "television" would be "tuh" or "tel," "nightly entertainment," or "My children watch too much _____" respectively. Mack was responsive to these types of cues and recognized immediately words he could not recall. While confrontation naming tasks had limited applicability to most of his life situations, some work in this area was also valuable. For example, he was asked to make a grocery list of items for a barbecue. And he enjoyed trying to come up with the names of family members, beers, and naming the kinds of ships in a navy fleet.

Interestingly, conversational speech was the most fruitful avenue for improving word retrieval skills. The reason for this was that Mack usually told his listener when he was having trouble finding a word rather than substitute another word, circumlocute, or change the subject. Early in treatment he "threw a fit" but subsequently he learned to cue the listener in more subtle ways. Sometimes he would stall for time. For example, when trying to say "Buick," he said "Let's see, what is it now, just a second." Sometimes, he produced a related word(s) which helped the listener focus on the desired word. When attempting to say "pen," he said "It's not a pencil." He could describe items he could not retrieve. For the word "checkers" he said "the game where there are 12 on one side and 12 on the other." Some of these problems resulted from production difficulties on multisyllabic words such as "detonator," but with effort he could self-correct these errors. Finally, there were occasions when he produced general labels such as "thing" and "it" in place of the desired word.

Transcriptions of Mack's conversational speech revealed that (a) he usually told his listener when he was having trouble, (b) he could provide some information about the word (e.g., description, related word), and (c) his efforts were inconsistently successful in "triggering" production of the desired word. To examine these phenomena more systematically, recordings of his conversational interactions in treatment were made and transcribed. Occurrences of word-finding difficulty were identified and the behaviors associated with each effort were categorized. Five categories of word retrieval behavior were delineated:

Delay: This involved taking or requesting additional time to produce the word. While some delay was inherent in all of Mack's retrieval efforts, he tended to use a filled pause, unfilled pause, or some stalling tactic to let me know he needed more time to produce the word.

Semantic Association: This entailed producing one or more words that were semantically related to the desired word. These include opposites (table-chair), in-class associations (Ford-Plymouth), part-whole relationships (branch-tree), and serially related items (Monday, Tuesday, Wednesday).

Phonetic Association: Mack produced a word or words that were phonetically similar to the desired word (patches, batches, matches.).

Description: He attempted to produce the desired word by describing what he was talking about (e.g., It's black and white).

Generalization: He emitted general words or what are termed empty words (thing, it, some) in place of the desired word.

The number of times Mack used these behaviors was counted and the percentage of times each behavior was followed by production of the desired word was calculated. Identifying the target word was relatively easy since Mack let the listener know this with exuberant gestures or statements like "I finally got that s.o.b."

Table 14.2 shows a distribution of Mack's word retrieval behaviors for the five categories, and the percentage of time each behavior was followed by the desired word. These data show that Mack used semantic association and description most often, and generalization and phonetic association the least. Delay, as a tactic, ranked in the middle. In terms of success, however, delay was the most successful behavior in "triggering" production of the desired word. Therefore, in treatment, Mack was encouraged to take more time in his word-retrieval efforts. This procedure involved letting him know he was having a problem and asking for more time. He did not stop using semantic association and description, but he was able to take some additional time after emitting these behaviors. This delaying tactic helped him elicit production of the desired word. Generalization seemed to be his way of letting the listener know the word was not readily available. In these rare instances, the word needed to be supplied for him.

TREATMENT COURSE

Changes in speech and language ability during treatment were objectively monitored with monthly administrations of the PICA. Mack's Overall percentile scores on the PICA during treatment and follow-up are shown in Figure 14.1. For the first three months of treatment he was seen twice weekly. He made modest gains and progressed from the

TABLE 14.2
Distribution of Client's Word Retrieval Behaviors and Percentage of Time Each Behavior "Triggered" Production of the Desired Word

BEHAVIOR	% USED	% SUCCESSFUL
Delay	23.2	89.4
Semantic Association	36.8	56.7
Phonetic Association	4.9	28.6
Description	24.9	52.1
Generalization	10.2	41.4

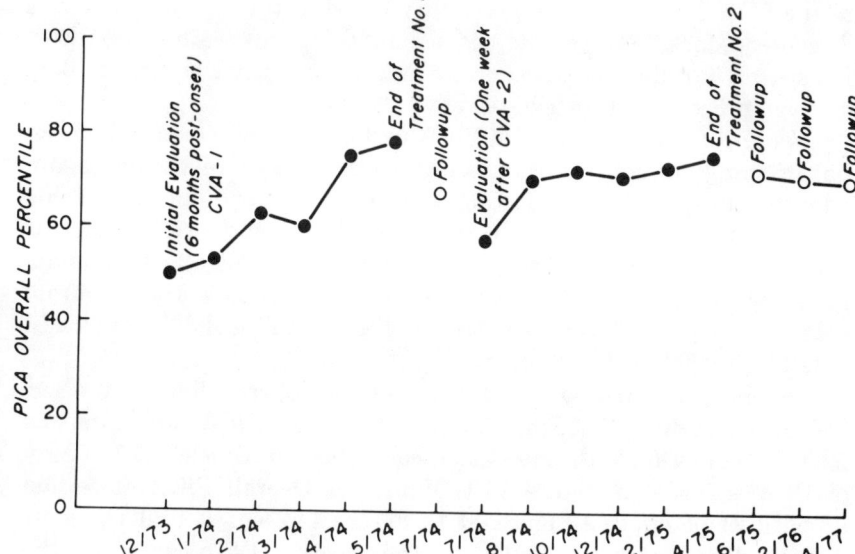

Figure 14.1 Overall percentile rankings on the PICA throughout Mack's treatment course.

49th to the 63rd percentile during the first two months, but after the third month of treatment, his PICA performance "sagged" slightly (60th percentile). This performance drop was attributed to his not getting enough treatment and the fact that he had missed some sessions due to bad weather.

Fortunately, Mack's mother lived near the VAMC. For the next month of treatment he moved into town and lived with her. His treatment time was increased from 2 to 10 sessions per week. This resulted in a marked increase in his Overall PICA score (60th to the 75th percentile). By this time his verbal communication had become quite functional, and he exhibited no observable problems in the comprehension of conversational speech. Reading was confined to the sports pages and headlines, but this was of interest to him. Writing remained severely limited and was abandoned as a therapeutic concern. Mack continued in treatment on a twice weekly basis for another month and eventually raised his overall PICA score to the 78th percentile. By this time he wanted to start playing golf again. A mutual decision was made to discontinue treatment and to see him monthly for follow-up.

Follow-up

In early July of 1974 Mack was seen for a follow-up visit. The PICA was readministered and he was found to have dropped from the 78th to the 67th percentile. The possibility of reinstituting treatment was discussed. Mack, however, did not feel anything was really wrong with his speech, but did express concern that he might not be able to play golf again because of his right-side weakness.

Second CVA. The drop in PICA performance was evidently a signal of things to come. Less than two weeks later, Mack was again admitted to the VAMC following a second CVA. The only noticeable neurological residual was an increased weakness on the right side, this time affecting the right lower extremity and adversely affecting ambulation. Mack was extremely depressed about this setback. He was afraid that he would keep having strokes and become an invalid; he expressed a desire "to die" if this occurred.

He was evaluated by speech-language pathology following the second insult on July 26, 1974. A comparison of his PICA subtest means for this evaluation with those attained at the end of treatment in May of 1974 is made in Figure 14.1. While his Overall PICA score had dropped 21 points (see Figure 14.1), Figure 14.2 shows that the most depressed subtest scores following the second CVA occurred on the writing tests, which had been nonfunctional at the conclusion of treatment in May 1974. Verbal scores (subtests I, IV, IX) except for repetition (XII) had decreased slightly, but still were relatively high. The impression was that Mack's potential for reestablishing functional verbal communication remained high in spite of the second stroke. Unfortunately, his depression, concern for physical limitations, and newly developed situations at home posed new challenges as he began for a second stint of treatment.

Treatment Following the Second CVA

Mack received one month of inpatient speech and language treatment. The first objective was to motivate him to communicate. This was accomplished by putting speech and language goals "on the back burner" and freeing his time to concentrate on more immediate needs, namely his ambulation. Speech and language treatment sessions were reduced so that Mack could spend more time in physical and occupational therapy. The physical and occupational therapists were counseled as to how best to communicate with him and given suggestions for providing language stimulation as they administered their treatments. His physician was consulted about the depression, and Mack was placed on antidepressant medications. After Mack had regained the ability to ambulate, speech and language treatment was provided once daily and generally followed the plan of treatment for the first CVA. Mack quickly progressed (Figure 14.1) from the 57th to the 70th percentile on the PICA. He was then discharged from the VAMC and seen on an outpatient basis.

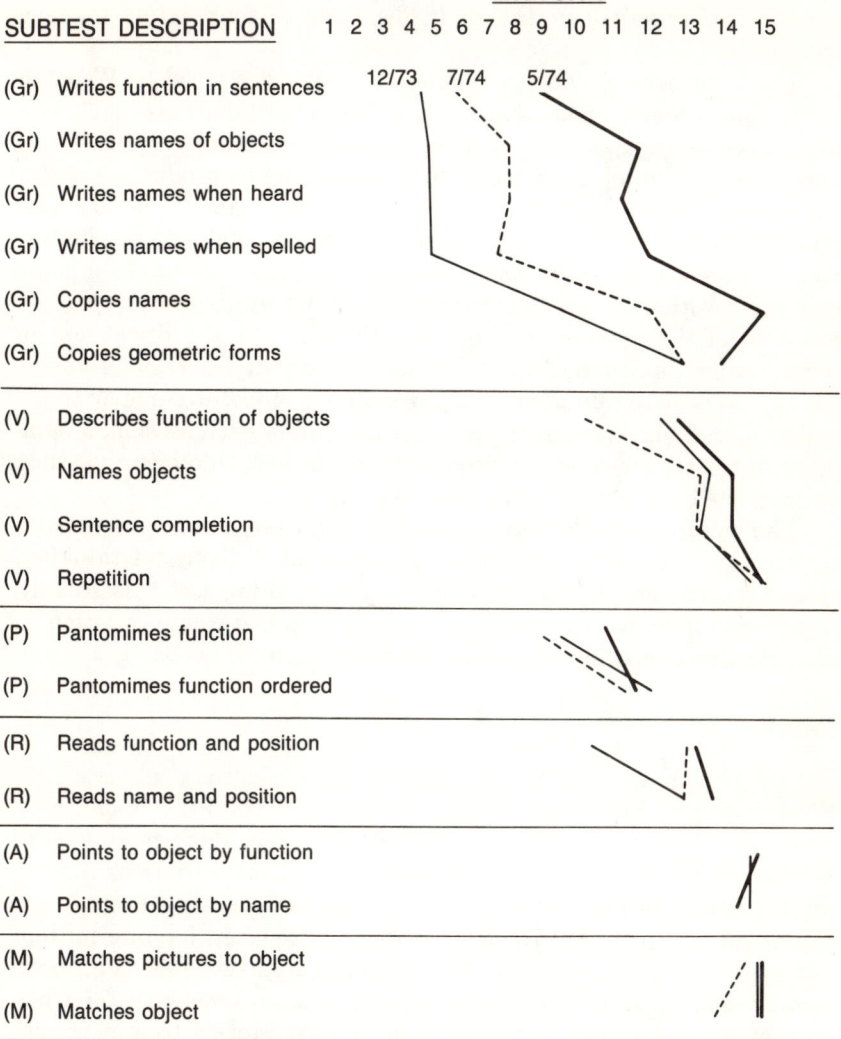

Figure 14.2 PICA subtest means for assessments after CVA 1 (5/73), after termination from treatment for CVA 1 (5/74), and after suffering CVA 2 (7/74).

Outpatient Treatment. After the second CVA, Mack needed strong supportive counseling and an opportunity to vent his feelings. Not only had he suffered a setback, but several stress producing situations had arisen in the home which necessitated his resuming a leadership role. His wife died after developing cancer. His two older children were having marital and employment problems, and his mother had passed away shortly after moving out of town and selling her home. These and other issues were imposed on the daily demands of four active teenage daughters.

The treatment provided was similar to that described by Wepman (1972) and recently elaborated upon by Martin (1981). This involved a thought-centered approach designed to stimulate thinking, flexibility, and to keep a flow of ideas going without dwelling on production of specific words. This focused on, as suggested by Searle (1967), "serious language." With Mack, it was seldom necessary to provide a topic; he had plenty of ideas of his own. As an example, he had never owned a home and was entitled to several benefits as a result of his military career. Substantial time was spent exploring the benefits and drawbacks of home ownership, financing, and other considerations. Other sessions focused on drawing up a will, the advisability of loaning money to his children, and alcohol consumption. At the end of each session, a summary of the topic(s) was prepared for him. He took this home to study and reported any action taken the following week.

The nondirected, client-centered approach gave Mack opportunities to function as speaker and listener; it stimulated divergent thinking, planning, problem solving, and helped him in making decisions. Finally, it provided a basis to continue to work to improve communication in real life situations that were directly relevant to his needs.

Results

Figure 14.1 shows that Mack maintained his treatment gains on the PICA following his second course of treatment. His PICA score, however, did not truly reflect his competency. At home, Mack reestablished his leadership role. He dealt effectively with many situations, including the deaths of his wife and mother. He was discharged from formal treatment in April of 1975. He continues to come in for intermittent follow-up visits, often calls on the phone, and participates in an occasional research project. PICA testing was discontinued in 1977 when he seemed to stabilize at the 70th percentile. Mack's treatment was successful. He maintained his gains and continues to do well today. He hopes for a new miracle surgery to "cure aphasia," but this does not dissuade him from working daily to improve himself.

REFERENCES

Brookshire, R.H. (1974). Differences in responding to auditory verbal materials among aphasic patients. *ACTA Symbolic,* 5, 1–18.
Darley, F.L. (1982). *Aphasia.* Philadelphia: W.B. Sanders.
DeRenzi, E., & Vignolo, L.A. (1962). The Token Test: A sensitive test to detect receptive disturbances in aphasics. *Brain,* 85, 665–678.

Dunn, L.M. (1965). *Peabody Picture Vocabulary Test.* Circle Pines. MN: American Guidance Service.

Goodglass, H., & Kaplan, E. (1972). *The assessment of aphasic and related disorders.* Philadelphia: Lea and Febiger.

Lezak, M.D. (1983). *Neuropsychological assessment.* New York: Oxford.

Liles, B.Z., & Brookshire, R.H. (1975). The effects of pause time on the auditory comprehension of aphasic subjects. *Journal of Communication Disorders, 8,* 221–231.

Martin, A.D. (1981). An examination of Wepman's thought centered therapy. In R. Chapey (Ed.), *Language intervention strategies in adult aphasia.* Baltimore: Williams & Wilkins.

Porch B.E. (1967). *Porch Index of Communicative Ability.* Palo Alto, CA: Consulting Psychologist.

Schuell, H. (1972). *The Minnesota Test for Differential Diagnosis of Aphasia.* Minneapolis: University of Minnesota Press.

Searle, J.R. (1967). *Speech acts: An essay in the philosophy of language.* New York: Cambridge University Press.

Wepman. J.M. (1972). Aphasia therapy: A new look. *Journal of Speech and Hearing Disorders, 37,* 203–214.

CHAPTER 15

Multiple Problems and Their Effect on Speech and Language Treatment

Thomas E. Prescott

> The aphasic client's course of speech and language treatment may be interrupted by several events, life-threatening or otherwise. Prescott describes the treatment course of a 68-year-old aphasic man who suffered two major medical setbacks. The clinical decision was to forge ahead with treatment and to continue to monitor change with periodic administrations of the PICA. Results indicated that the client continued to progress in spite of his setbacks.

1. What background information does Prescott provide that suggests the client may have been prone to suffering multiple strokes? What are the prognostic ramifications?
2. List some of the behavioral characteristics documented by the author that suggested that the client was improving in treatment. How might these changes be measured on the PICA? In other ways?
3. Give the steps of the "verbing" program used to treat this client. What is Prescott's rationale for using this approach?
4. The PICA was administered periodically to document treatment change. Does this procedure have any advantages? Any disadvantages?

INTRODUCTION

The road to recovery from aphasia is not always smooth. The patient may suffer medical setbacks, personal crises, and encounter other obstacles that alter or slow his treatment course. Paul, a 68-year-old aphasic man seen at the Denver VA Medical Center, traveled such a road. He suffered two major medical events during his course of aphasia treatment. The first was right-hemisphere CVA which terminated speech and language treatment for nearly six months; the second was cancer with its impending fear of death. Following each complication, the clinician had to refocus treatment, adjust treatment goals, and continue treatment to prevent the patient from losing ground. Ongoing documentation of treatment indicated that Paul continued to progress in spite of his medical difficulties.

THE CASE: PAUL

Medical History

Paul, a 68-year-old retired barber, had a 15-year history of transient ischemic attacks (TIAs), hypertension (controlled by medication), and diabetes (controlled by diet). He was married and the father of four grown children. On September 23, 1982, Paul was brought by his wife to the emergency room complaining of a sudden onset of right-sided weakness and inability to speak. Over the course of an hour his motor deficits partially resolved, but his speech and language deficits remained essentially unchanged.

Because the patient's motor deficits had resolved so rapidly, his initial medical diagnosis was that he had probably suffered another TIA. On the next day he was reexamined by a neurologist, and a CT scan of the head without contrast was performed. A neurologic exam revealed that Paul's motor deficits had totally resolved, but some mild sensory deficits remained, and he was still having difficulty with his speech. The CT scan revealed some brain atrophy with no indication of recent infarction or bleeding. At this time, the diagnosis was changed from that of a TIA to one of a completed stroke.

SPEECH AND LANGUAGE EVALUATION

Paul was informally evaluated by the speech-language pathologist the day after his CVA. It was evident that he had improved markedly in one day's time, but his language and speech were still significantly impaired. He communicated with single words (content words) and short phrases. Many of these utterances contained literal (foon/spoon) and verbal (car/bus) paraphasic errors. Paul could name items presented by the examiner 50% of the time, and he could point to items named by the examiner in the room 60% of the time. On longer messages such as two-part commands (e.g., Point to the window and the chair), he had more difficulties, often needing a repetition of the stimulus before he could respond.

On October 20, 1982, one month postonset, the *Porch Index of Communicative Ability* (PICA) (Porch, 1967) was administered. Paul attained an overall mean score of 11.59, placing him at the 59th percentile in a large random sample of left-hemisphere damaged adults. Corresponding percentile rankings for the Gestural, Verbal, and Graphic modalities were the 57th, 52nd, and 68th percentiles respectively (see Table 15.1 and Figure 15.1). On the PICA, he demonstrated an across-the-board impairment in all language modalities. The major determinant of success or failure on a given task was the difficulty of the task in question. For example, he made few errors on the easy subtests of the PICA (matching and copying). He had more difficulty with the naming, reading, and pantomime subtests on the PICA but still performed relatively well. Pronounced problems were evident on the more difficult PICA tests (writing and sentence formulation).

Prognosis

At one month postonset Paul appeared to be an excellent candidate for speech and language treatment. He had exhibited high motivation to improve his communication from the onset of his stroke, and his spontaneous recovery was good. His predicted target percentile for the PICA at six months postonset using the HOAP slope formula devised by Porch (1971) was the 90th percentile. More important, Paul exhibited behaviors that reflected an awareness of his difficulties and an emerging

TABLE 15.1
Test Data

DATE	NORMS	OVERALL	GESTURAL	VERBAL	GRAPHIC
10/20/82	Left brain damaged	59	57	52	68
11/22/82	Left brain damaged	77	78	77	77
01/15/83	Left brain damaged	79	81	76	79
06/07/83	Bilateral	86	84	82	86
07/07/83	Bilateral	89	90	92	88
08/18/83	Bilateral	90	94	92	86
09/22/83	Bilateral	99	99	99	85

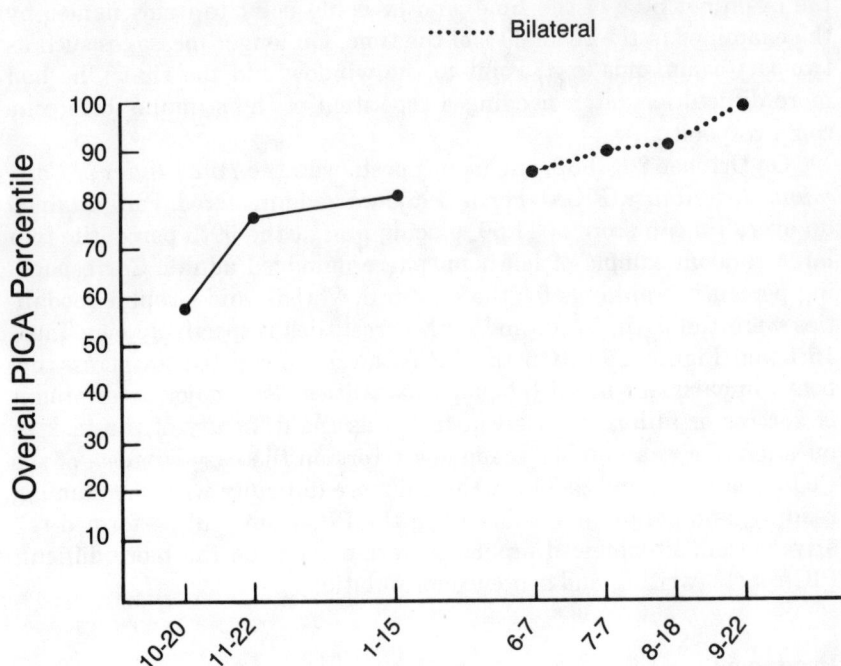

Figure 15.1 Overall PICA percentile rankings throughout the patient's treatment course. Left hemisphere norms were used after the first (left) CVA. Bilateral norms were employed after his second (right) CVA.

ability to compensate for them. For example, he asked for repeats if he did not understand. These auditory processing problems resulted from what has been termed noise build-up (Brookshire, 1972; Porch, 1967). On structured tasks, this was seen as a breakdown in comprehension after every fourth or fifth item in a series. This noise build-up could be overcome by giving Paul 10 to 20 second rest periods every four or five responses. Paul tended to repeat (reauditorize) instructions on auditory tasks. This propensity for repetition seemed to help him process the message (when his repetitions were accurate). However, when his repetitions were inaccurate, his comprehension was similarly deleteriously affected in that he usually responded inaccurately.

TREATMENT

Paul was seen for speech and language treatment five times per week beginning October 21, 1982. Treatment focused on improving auditory processing beginning with simple tasks such as identifying alphabet letters and following one-step commands (e.g., Touch your chin) and progressing systematically to more difficult tasks such as two-stage commands (e.g., Before you point to the window, snap your fingers). Paul was encouraged to use self-imposed time-outs to maintain performance accuracy on auditory comprehension tasks. Writing was introduced using a simple dictation task in which the clinician spelled highly useful words for Paul (e.g., M-I-L-K) and he wrote the word. In this first month of treatment, Paul was also introduced to a "verbing" treatment program developed by Loverso, Selinger, and Prescott (1979).

"Verbing" Program. The "verbing" program is intended to elicit two levels of responses from the patient. Level I tasks require a subject + verb sentence (e.g., The boy is running), and Level II tasks require a subject + verb + object construction (e.g., The boy is eating cake). If the subject is unable to function at either Level I or Level II, prelevels (IA, IB and IIA, IIB) are introduced requiring easier performance tasks initially and gradually increasing in difficulty in preparation for the next level. In conducting the program, the clinician shows the patient an action picture, and cues him to produce the subject with a "Wh" question (e.g., Who is running?). A similar tactic is employed to elicit the object (e.g., What is the boy eating?). All tasks in the "verbing" program are aimed at providing the patient with a self-cueing strategy to ameliorate his word-finding difficulties. In addition, the program provides practice in a structured setting. Thompson and Kearns (1981) conducted a study wherein they evaluated the acquisition, generalization, and maintenance of naming behavior in a patient with anomia. These authors concluded that the patient was able to learn and to maintain over time a period of acquired naming but was unable to generalize to untrained names. In 1982, Prescott, Selinger, and Loverso demonstrated similar effects with verbs except that the learning that occurred generalized to untrained verbs. The "verbing" program, therefore, appeared to be a usable treatment approach and a functional communication strategy.

After One Month

Paul made remarkable gains in the first month of treatment. These changes were seen behaviorally, and by his scores in the readministration of the PICA. His Overall mean score on the PICA of 13.05 (see Table 15.1 and Figure 15.1) placed him at the 77th percentile and represented a marked improvement from the previous month. Similar gains were seen in the Gestural, Verbal, and Graphic modalities on the PICA in treatment and in formal testing. Paul needed far fewer repetitions, and while many of his responses were delayed, they were usually accurate. It appeared as if he was well on his way to achieving and perhaps surpassing his six-month target percentile (90th percentile) for the PICA. The second month of treatment began on this optimistic note.

As treatment continued, Paul's accuracy on all tasks continued to increase. His ability to attend to auditory stimuli and to take self-imposed rest breaks when his system became overloaded improved his comprehension to a point where this was not a problem for him in functional situations. He independently slowed his speech rate and took the time to self-correct his errors. The clinician seldom needed to remind him to make these compensations. As he improved his performance on the "verbing" program his speech became increasingly fluent and his output increased. At this time he also began to work on his defective reading skills by completing homework assignments from Level D of the *Specific Skill Series, Getting the Main Ideas and Using the Context* (Boning, 1976). Performance on these homework assignments was monitored using the Base 10 scoring forms developed by LaPointe (1979). Data accumulated in the second month of treatment indicated that progress was being made.

After Two Months

Aphasic patients seen regularly for treatment are usually tested monthly with a standardized test battery. In Paul's case, this entailed monthly administration of the PICA. As the end of Paul's second month of treatment neared, he began to miss some treatment sessions due to illness. The PICA could not be administered again until January 15, 1983, nearly two months after his last test. At this time (see Table 15.1 and Figure 15.1) Paul attained an Overall mean score of 13.17, placing him at the 79th percentile; his gains on the Gestural and Verbal subtests were negligible. Evidently, these minimal improvements on the PICA from prior testing were signals of things to come. Paul was readmitted to the hospital the next day after suffering a second CVA, this time involving the right hemisphere.

REENTERING TREATMENT

Following his right-hemisphere CVA, Paul spent time in the hospital and nursing home and had a lengthy convalesent period at home. He received no speech and language treatment for almost six months. He was reevaluated as a candidate for treatment in June of 1983. At this time he achieved an Overall mean score on the PICA (see Table 15.1 and Figure 15.1) of 12.75 which placed him at the 73rd percentile in a large random sample of left-hemisphere damaged adults. It is noteworthy that this score approximated that for his evaluation the day before the onset of the right-hemisphere CVA, but since there was a six-month gap between the insult and readministration of the PICA, it cannot be determined if Paul's performance at this time reflects regaining of lost ground or maintenance of the status quo. Since Paul had now suffered left- and right-hemisphere insults, it was no longer appropriate to monitor his performance on the PICA with the left-hemisphere norms. Fortunately, Porch (1971) has also provided normative data on the PICA for bilaterally involved patients. Paul's Overall mean score on the PICA placed him at the 86th percentile on the bilateral norms (see Table 15.1 and Figure 15.1). Corresponding performance levels using the bilateral norms were similarly elevated for the modality means.

Paul was administered some additional testing as he reentered treatment. These included the *Revised Token Test* (RRT) (McNeil & Prescott, 1978) and the *Reading Comprehension Battery for Aphasia* (RCBA) (LaPointe & Horner, 1979). RTT results suggested that his auditory processing performance was now adversely affected by stimulus length and linguistic complexity. Reading performance reflected similar deficits. He did well at the single word level but had problems comprehending longer units requiring inferential thinking and processing of morpho-syntactic constructions. His writing and verbal abilities reflected similar types of problems as well as word-retrieval difficulties. Paul retained the ability to self-correct many of his production errors.

As Paul reentered treatment, a new set of objectives was formulated. These included (a) improving auditory comprehension within conversational interactions, (b) increasing quantity and complexity of verbal output to produce more syntactically complete sentences, (c) increasing word retrieval skills at the word and sentence level, (d) improving reading at the paragraph level, and (e) improving sentence writing ability.

Close procedures were employed to assist Paul in retrieving specific words on short-answer and sentence level tasks. This involved spoken and written sentence completion tasks (e.g., The Denver weather is __). and paragraph reading. The clinician had Paul read paragraphs in which several key content words were missing. Paul's job was to fill in the missing words so that the paragraph read logically. Similar procedures were employed to enhance written word retrieval except that Paul was required to read the paragraph and write in the missing elements. He worked on several tasks designed to stimulate what Chapey (1981) has called convergent and divergent thinking. The former included tasks such as category recall (e.g., Name as many NFL teams as you can) and supplying synonyms, antonyms, and homonyms. The latter involved production tasks to elicit a variety of responses such as "List all the possible uses you can think of for a piece of glass," or "Tell me all the things that might happen to you while eating lunch at a restaurant," and responding to an array of "Wh" questions (e.g., "What would happen if you spilled your milk?"). Task instructions for these activities required Paul to work on improving his auditory processing skills as well.

Reentry, After One Month

Paul continued to benefit from speech and language treatment after his second CVA. PICA results (see Table 15.1 and Figure 15.1) one month (July 7, 1983) after reentering treatment reflected general across-the-board gains in all areas tested. Readministration of the RTT revealed an improvement in auditory processing skills. Paul now understood RRT commands of greater length and complexity than on prior testing.

It was at this time that Paul suffered a second medical setback. He was found to have cancer of the prostate. Medical management for this life-threatening condition superseded his need for speech and language treatment, and his treatment sessions were reduced from five times per week to two times per week.

Reentry, After Two Months

Paul came to treatment on a reduced schedule for another month. Treatment goals and activities remained largely unchanged. Again Paul improved. PICA results (see Table 15.1 and Figure 15.1) using bilateral norms revealed consistent gains (August 18, 1983). In addition, Paul's wife reported that he was communicating effectively in situations outside the clinic. Since he had continued to progress at a time when treatment time was reduced, another month of treatment was planned.

In the next month Paul completed units IV through XII in the *Specific Skill Series Booklet B, Locating the Answer* (Boning, 1976) with 100% accuracy. Although he did well providing responses to convergent tasks, his ability to read and comprehend material requiring divergent thinking was variable (50% to 80% success). In short, he did better with specific detail questions than on those necessitating broad answers. Paul's writing also lacked syntactic complexity, and spelling errors were abundant in his written efforts. In what was to be his final month of treatment, Paul was provided a list of words of high personal interest to him, and he worked on learning to spell these words. With great effort he improved to a point where he could spell 60% to 70% of his key words correctly.

Reentry, After Three Months, and Termination

The possibility of termination from treatment was approached with Paul three months after he began treatment for his second CVA. The PICA was readministered (see Table 15.1 and Figure 15.1). Results indicated the patient had reached the 99th percentile on the bilateral norms for his Overall, Gestural, and Verbal mean scores; Graphic performance was at the 85th percentile. To gain an appreciation of how he might be using language in more functional settings, Paul was also given the *Communicative Abilities in Daily Living* (CADL) (Holland, 1980). Out of a total of 136 possible points, Paul attained a score of 115. This performance is below the CADL mean for normal subjects on an equivalent age (127.70) but well above the mean score for aphasic subjects in the same age range (97.60). Since his performance, on both functional and more formalized measures were highly correlated, and his wife continued to indicate that his communication was highly functional in situations within and outside of the home, treatment was terminated.

SUMMARY

Paul's treatment was considered to have been warranted and highly successful in spite of two medically significant events. When he began treatment following a left-hemisphere CVA, he progressed rapidly over a two-month period. After stopping treatment because of a right-hemisphere stroke, having no treatment for six months, he reentered treatment and continued to improve for three additional months. Monitoring Paul's treatment progress with continued administrations of the PICA, first using left-hemisphere norms, then bilateral norms, permitted the clinician to chart progress, redefine goals and procedures, and come to a decision as to when treatment should end.

The results of this man's treatment are like life—difficult and sometimes surprising. Intervening variables such as second strokes, illness, and other crises create difficult decisions for busy clinicians. The decision in the case presented here was to "push on" and continue treatment. The progress made in spite of Paul's medical setbacks suggests that our work does some good.

The procedures used in Paul's treatment are not given as "the way" to treat aphasia, but instead to provide an example of one attempt to treat a patient with aphasia.

REFERENCES

Boning, R.A. (1976). *Specific skill series: Getting the main idea.* Book E. Baldwin, NY: Barnell Loft.

Boning, R.A. (1976). *Specific skill series: Using the context.* Book E. Baldwin, NY: Barnell Loft.

Boning, R.A. (1976). *Specific skill series: Locating the answer.* Book D. Baldwin, NY: Barnell Loft.

Brookshire, R.H. (1972, November). *Differences in auditory processing deficits among aphasic patients.* Paper presented to the Annual Convention of American Speech and Hearing Association, San Francisco.

Chapey, R. (1981). Divergent semantic interaction. In R. Chapey (Ed.), *Language intervention strategies in adult aphasia.* Baltimore: Williams & Wilkins.

Holland, A.L. (1981). *Communicative Abilities in Daily Living.* Austin, TX: PRO-ED.

LaPointe, L.L. (1979). *Base 10 response form.* Tigard, OR: C.C. Publications.

LaPointe, L.L., & Horner, J. (1979). *Reading Comprehension Battery for Aphasia.* Tigard. OR: C.C. Publications.

Loverso, F.L., Selinger, M., & Prescott. T.E. (1979). Application of verbing strategies to aphasia treatment. In R. Brookshire (Ed.), *Clinical Aphasiology Conference Proceedings.* Minneapolis: BRK Publishers.

McNeil, M.R., & Hageman, C.F. (1979). Auditory processing deficits in aphasia evidenced on the Revised Token Test. In R. Brookshire (Ed.), *Clinical Aphasiology Conference Proceedings.* Minneapolis: BRK Publishers.

McNeil, M.R., & Prescott. T.E. (1978). *The Revised Token Test.* Austin, TX: PRO-ED.

Porch, B.E. (1967). *Porch Index of Communicative Ability.* Palo Alto, CA: Consulting Psychologists Press.

Porch, B.E. (1971). *Porch Index of Communicative Ability, Vol. II: Administration, Scoring, Interpretation* (rev. ed.). Palo Alto, CA: Consulting Psychologists Press.

Prescott. T.E., Selinger, M., & Loverso, F.L. (1982). An analysis of learning, generalization, and maintenance of verbs by an aphasic patient. In R. Brookshire (Ed.), *Clinical Aphasiology Conference Proceedings.* Minneapolis: BRK Publishers.

Thompson, C., & Kearns, K.P. (1981). An experimental analysis of acquisition, generalization, and maintenance of naming behavior in a patient with anomia. In R. Brookshire (Ed.), *Clinical Aphasiology Conference Proceedings.* Minneapolis: BRK Publishers.

CHAPTER 16
Systematic Programming of Verbal Elaboration Skills in Chronic Broca's Aphasia
Kevin P. Kearns

> Kearns provides an excellent example of how a within-subject experimental design can be used in aphasia treatment. He reports the results of a program designed to facilitate elaborated spontaneous verbal responses by a client with chronic Broca's aphasia. The author demonstrates how scientifically acceptable methods can be used to measure treatment effects and generalization. Significantly, Kearns' treatment focuses on communicative function rather than eliciting preselected target responses by "loosening" patient response requirements during training.
>
> 1. What evidence does the author give to indicate the patient had plateaued in previous treatment? Why did Kearns reinstitute treatment with this client?
> 2. How do the "loose" training strategies as described by Kearns differ from the manner in which aphasia treatment is usually conducted? What advantages do these strategies have in enhancing the patient's communicative functioning?
> 3. Review carefully the author's procedures for making baseline measures, defining acceptable responses, clinical probe measures, and scoring responses. What importance do these procedures have in determining the effects of the treatment provided?

Introduction

A philosophy of aphasia management which emphasizes communicative function over linguistic form has emerged in recent years (Holland, 1977; Davis & Wilcox, 1981). Consistent with this philosophy has been the development of training approaches based on pragmatic and interactive aspects of communication. The movement away from structural aspects of language and renewed interest in communication per se can be seen, in part, as a reaction to the use of overly structured training techniques. Frequently, the content of aphasia treatment is didactic and unidirectional with an emphasis on eliciting responses from the patient (Davis & Wilcox, 1981). In addition, there may be a stubborn insistence on the part of clinicians that there is only one acceptable response to the treatment task, the one selected by the clinician. Although language and communication are used creatively and with great flexibility in the natural environment, overly didactic training approaches can inhibit the patient's creative use of language and communication by restricting the patient responses. Similarly, clinicians may extinguish or even punish creative language use by ignoring or admonishing novel but appropriate patient responses when overly structured treatment approaches are employed.

It is, perhaps, no surprise that many aphasic patients become "cue bound" and fail to generalize newly acquired skills to nontraining settings when we insist that they respond in the predetermined manner of our choice. Stokes and Baer (1977) have suggested that overly structured training techniques may inhibit generalization by training clients to discriminate treatment conditions from other settings and conditions in which generalization might be expected. To overcome the deleterious effects of overly structured training, they suggest varying the stimulus, response, and feedback conditions within therapy sessions. By sampling a wider range of conditions in treatment, it is less likely that patients will restrict their responses to the treatment setting. Consistent with these "loose training" suggestions, techniques emphasizing patient initiated responses and reinforcing creative language, instead of demanding specific target responses, may facilitate generative responding from our aphasic patients.

Although "loose training" programs are not available for the aphasic population, Hart (1981) and Hart and Risley (1974) have developed such a program for remediation of language problems in preschool children. Their "incidental teaching" approach is carried out in the preschool environment rather than in a treatment room. It was developed after Hart observed that overly structured, didactic approaches did not effectively alter communication in the natural environment. One important element of Hart's novel incidental teaching approach is that the clinician shapes and elaborates spontaneously produced client responses rather than targeting responses which are preselected by the clinician. Of equal importance, the communicative success of patient-initiated responses are given priority over the specific linguistic structures as a means of communicating. Hart's incidental teaching approach demonstrates that a pragmatic philosophy of language training can be combined with intervention techniques such as modeling, prompting, and social reinforcement to obtain generative responding in language-delayed children. Needless to say, programs that translate a pragmatic philosophy of language intervention into practical training techniques are also needed for our aphasic patients.

Purpose

The following study demonstrates one method of combining the treatment philosophy outlined above with a data-based treatment approach. The specific purpose of this clinical study was to evaluate the effectiveness of a response elaboration training technique for a patient with chronic Broca's aphasia. The treatment program was applied to patient-initiated responses in an attempt to increase the amount of information that is spontaneously provided (i.e., number of "content" words) during a picture description task. Generalization of more elaborate responding to familiar, untrained stimuli was also explored.

THE CASE: MIKE

Patient Description

Mike is a 50-year-old man who experienced a sudden onset of right-sided hemiplegia and aphasia on April 19, 1981. The medical diagnosis at the time of his admission to the hospital was thrombosis of the left middle cerebral artery. He had a history of hypertension, but his medical history was otherwise unremarkable. Mike was a recent widower, and following his discharge from the hospital he returned home where he lived with his mother and two sons, ages 7 and 23. He completed grade school and is a former longshoreman.

Mike was referred to the New Orleans VA Medical Center speech pathology department on June 26, 1981, approximately two months after his cerebrovascular accident. *The Porch Index of Communicative Abilities* (PICA) (Porch, 1967) was administered to assess his residual speech and language skills, and the following results were obtained:

Date	Overall Percentile	Gestural Percentile	Verbal Percentile	Graphic Percentile
6/26/81	7.03–18	10.44–23	2.00–1	5.84–23

The Overall PICA score of 7.03 and the results across Gestural, Verbal, and Graphic subtests revealed a severe aphasic deficit affecting all language modalities. Mike was mute. He did not verbalize or vocalize during the entire evaluation, and additional testing revealed a severe oral-verbal apraxia.

Treatment History

Following his initial evaluation Mike was enrolled in both individual and group treatment. Individual sessions were held twice weekly for about one hour, and a one-hour group session was conducted weekly. Attendance in treatment was consistently good from July 1981 until August 1983. Although additional treatment was scheduled from August 1983 to December 1983, attendance was poor during this period because of minor illnesses and vacations. Multimodality stimulation was provided during treatment, and individual goals were established to meet the patient's specific needs. Initial goals included improvement of auditory comprehension ability and development of a functional gestural communication system (Skelly, 1979). Treatment tasks were also designed to reduce the severity of oral-verbal apraxia and improve verbal skills.

Periodic administration of the PICA throughout the period of intervention demonstrated consistent improvement. Selected test results are shown below to highlight Mike's progress in treatment.

Date	Overall Percentile	Gestural Percentile	Verbal Percentile	Graphic Percentile
6/81	7.03–18	10.44–23	2.00– 1	5.84–23
6/82	10.17–46	12.66–49	9.10–42	7.55–50
6/83	10.52–49	12.73–50	9.98–45	7.93–55

In general, from the time of the initial test evaluation in June of 1981 until his final examination at the end of regular attendance at treatment two years later, performance improved from an Overall score of 7.03 (18% percentile) to an Overall score of 10.52 (49% percentile). Improvement was also evident across all modalities with the most dramatic gains apparent for verbal performance.

As previously noted, Mike did not attend treatment regularly between June and December of 1983. He was, however, retested with the PICA in December, 1983, to determine if he had plateaued on formal testing and had maintained previous treatment gains. As shown in the following table, readministration of the PICA revealed negligible differences between results of testing at the end of regular treatment and performance on followup testing.

Date	Overall Percentile	Gestural Percentile	Verbal Percentile	Graphic Percentile
6/83	10.52–49	12.73–50	9.98–45	7.93–55
12/83	10.65–50	13.38–66	9.58–44	7.75–53

In general, it appeared that Mike's performance on the PICA had plateaued. Although a change was apparent on his Gestural performance, differences between posttreatment Gestural scores (12.73) and Gestural performance on the follow-up test (13.38) were not felt to be clinically significant. Overall, he maintained the level of performance exhibited on formal testing at the end of regular attendance in treatment for a period of six months prior to the start of this experimental treatment program.

At the time of retesting Mike exhibited a moderately severe Broca's aphasia and a mild to moderate verbal apraxia. His speech was telegraphic. That is, spontaneous utterances usually consisted of one or two content words (nouns, verbs, etc.) while functors (auxiliary verbs, articles, etc.) and grammatical endings were frequently deleted. Apractic errors, primarily phoneme substitutions and distortions, occurred, but the majority of Mike's one and two word responses were intelligible in context. Speech initiation difficulties and some "struggle" behaviors were also evident.

As one would expect for a patient with Broca's aphasia, Mike's auditory comprehension was functional for everyday conversation (PICA VI, $\overline{X}$ = 14.4; PICA X, $\overline{X}$ = 14.6). His graphic output remained nonfunctional and consisted primarily of legible, incorrect strings of letters.

A Rationale for Continued Treatment

Although Mike had plateaued on formal testing and had received a considerable amount of treatment, several factors mitigated against his dismissal from treatment. For example, despite a heavy emphasis on verbal tasks, he seldom spontaneously initiated a communicative interaction, and his responses to direct questions or requests consisted primarily of one and two word utterances. Moreover, he rarely attempted to elaborate on a point of conversation. When encouraged to provide more information, he typically responded, "I don't know, I don't know." Since he supplied a limited amount of information to those who interacted with him, listeners often guessed what Mike was attempting to communicate, and this further fragmented communication. He did use a wide variety of functional gestures, but the information supplied through gestures was often redundant with his verbal output. In general, he did not actively share the "burden of communication," and his ability to initiate and maintain an interaction was limited.

Several other factors were also considered in deciding whether further treatment was warranted for Mike. Namely, he was young and highly motivated to continue treatment and he had a supportive family. Significantly, he was attempting to maintain his role as the head of the family despite his language impairment. After reviewing all relevant factors, it was decided that a final period of additional treatment was warranted.

Goal of Treatment

From a functional viewpoint, Mike's language skills far surpassed his communication abilities. In particular, his lack of initiation and reduced responsiveness severely limited his opportunity for communicative interaction. Moreover, his clinician felt that the didactic, structured verbal treatment approaches that had previously been used with Mike might have contributed to his decreased responsiveness. Therefore, a within-subject experimental design was used to evaluate the effectiveness and generalization of a response-elaboration training program that "loosened" the structure of treatment.

The goal of treatment was to facilitate an increase in the amount of information spontaneously provided by Mike in response to simple action pictures. The emphasis in training was on combining successive, patient initiated responses until more elaborate spontaneous descriptions were achieved.

Materials

The materials used for training in this study consisted of 30 black and white line drawings depicting transitive and intransitive verbs (see Appendix A). The 5×4-inch action cards were taken from commercially available materials (Fokes, 1976), and each showed an individual engaged in an unambiguous action such as running or throwing. Although the purchased materials had a target verb printed on the front of each stimulus card, the printing was removed from the stimulus cards used in this study.

The thirty line drawings were divided into three sets of 10 items each. Two sets were designated as training items and the third set was used to probe generalization. The ten items in the generalization set were included because Mike had previously been exposed to these items during treatment. Given his familiarity with these items, it was felt that any improvements evident on the training items might carry over to the generalization items. He had never been exposed to the two sets of training items prior to his participation in this study.

The setting for this study was a clinic room in the speech pathology section of the New Orleans VA Medical Center. During training and baseline sessions the clinician was seated to the right of Mike and both were seated in front of a treatment table. Sessions were scheduled three times weekly and each session lasted for approximately 40 minutes. Only the clinician and patient were in the room during experimental sessions. A Morantz Superscope audio cassette recorder was used to tape record each session. Tapes were later analyzed for accuracy of transcription, and the transcribed responses were rescored by an independent observer for reliability purposes.

EXPERIMENTAL DESIGN

A multiple-baseline design across behaviors was used in this study (McReynolds & Kearns, 1983). There are two primary phases of a multiple baseline study, the baseline phase and the treatment phase. Baseline (A) refers to a period of testing during which the patient's level of responding is measured prior to the initiation of treatment. During the treatment phase (B) an experimental treatment program is administered. In a multiple baseline study, treatment is sequentially applied to one of several similar but independent groups of responses while baseline testing continues on the remaining groups of responses. Using this design, treatment effectiveness is demonstrated when improvement occurs for training responses only, and minimal changes are observed for other sets of responses that have not been directly trained. As subsequent sets of responses are sequentially trained, the responses being treated should improve while the remaining, untreated sets of responses should not change significantly. A strong correlation between improvement in performance when treatment is applied to a set of responses and absence of change in performance prior to treatment provides convincing evidence that training is effective.

Baseline

During each session of the baseline (A) phase, the thirty stimulus items were randomized and individually presented. The initial baseline sessions were conducted within one week of the initiation of training on the first set of items. Baseline sessions were introduced with the general instruction, "I am going to show you some pictures and I want you to tell me as much as you can about them." Upon presentation of the first item, the clinician also said, "As completely as possible, tell me about this picture." The instruction was repeated if Mike requested a repetition, if he did not respond within approximately fifteen seconds, or if an unintelligible, perseverative, irrelevant, or stereotypic response occurred. He was given as much time as needed to describe the stimulus item. The trial ended and a second item was placed before him when he indicated (gesturally or verbally) that he had finished his description of the first item, or after he was silent for approximately fifteen seconds. Instructions were not repeated prior to presenting the remaining items unless the previously noted conditions for repetition were met. Furthermore, contingent feedback and reinforcement were not provided during the baseline phase.

Response Definition and Scoring. The primary measure of improvement in this study was the number of content words produced by Mike in response to each of the stimulus pictures. Relevant content words were tallied and the number of content words per response were calculated for baseline and clinical probes. All appropriate nouns, pronouns, main verbs, adjectives, adverbs, and prepositions were credited as a single content word. Alternately, auxiliary verbs, articles and grammatical endings (e.g., *-ing, -ed*) were not tallied in this study. Perseverative or stereotypic utterances and unintelligible responses were also not tallied in the scoring system. Reiterative utterances (e.g., "wash, wash, wash") and multiple repetitions of the same word in a single response were counted as a single content word. Mike was not penalized for minor articulatory errors as long as the target word was clearly intelligible in context. For example, a /w/ for /r/ substitution was acceptable for the word "running" in response to the stimulus item that depicted that action.

Since the purpose of this study was to facilitate response elaboration or "creative language," content words did not have to be depicted in a stimulus action card to be tallied as long as the information conveyed was clearly relevant for that item. For example, in response to a picture of a person running Mike stated, "Man . . . running . . . bus" on one occasion and "bus . . . left him" on another occasion. In both instances, a score of three content words was recorded even though there was no bus or bus stop depicted on the stimulus item.

Clinical Probes. Following the original baseline phase, baseline testing continued on alternate days when treatment was not scheduled to occur. These "clinical probes" were used as the primary measure of progress in this study. Procedures used during the administration and scoring of clinical probes were identical to those used during baseline.

Treatment Phase

The treatment phase of the study began following the third baseline session. During the treatment phase the two sets of training items were individually and sequentially trained to criterion. Initially, the first set was trained and training was withheld for the second set. Training was initiated on the second set of items after the first set had been trained to criterion. The criterion for terminating training for both sets of items was production of five or more content words in response to at least eight of ten training items during clinical probes. The study ended after the second set of training items was trained to criterion. Generalization items were never trained during this investigation.

Treatment Program. Individual treatment sessions consisted of two random presentations of a set of training items. A five minute break was allowed between the first and second presentation of the training set. Although each session was tape recorded for reliability purposes, on-line transcription was used to help the clinician follow the treatment protocol. That is, the clinician wrote down each content word produced by the patient at each step in a training trial to ensure appropriate use of modeling and cueing during treatment.

Each trial during a treatment session involved a sequence of steps designed to facilitate more elaborate patient responding. Patient-initiated utterances were modified through modeling, shaping, and chaining techniques. Mike's responses were expanded to include more content words by reinforcing the use of novel, appropriate utterances and by systematically combining newly supplied information with previous content. Clinician expansion of patient responses was kept to a minimum, and Mike was prompted to provide additional information that could be added to earlier descriptions of the stimulus pictures. Although the training techniques were both systematic and highly structured, they were designed to facilitate interaction between the clinician and patient by allowing an exchange of old and new information. A training trial consisted of completing the six step sequence twice for a given training item. The six steps in the training sequence are outlined in Table 16.1.

Treatment sessions began with the instruction, "I'm going to show you some pictures and I want you to tell me as much as you can about them." The first training trial began when an item was placed in front of Mike and he was instructed, "As completely as possible, tell me about this picture." A repetition of this Step 1 instruction was provided if an unintelligible, perseverative, or stereotypic response was produced, or if Mike asked for a repetition. A repetition was also allowed at subsequent steps in the program if an appropriate response was not elicited or if a repetition of an instruction was requested. For example, the step was repeated if an unintelligible response was produced at steps 3 or 5 in the program. In addition, these steps were repeated if Mike did not provide an appropriate elaboration (step 3) or imitation (step 5) upon request.

An elaboration was defined as any response that contained one or more relevant content words that had not been provided during the

Table 16.1
Elaboration of Patient Initiated Responses

Step	Clinician	Patient
1	Verbal instruction and stimulus presentation.	Spontaneous Description. For example, "Crying"
2	Expansion, model, reinforce, for example "A man is crying. Good.	No response.
3	"Wh" Cue. For example, "*Why* is he crying?"	Elaboration. For example, "Hit head"
4	Combine patient responses, model, reinforce. For example, "Great. The man is crying because he hit his head."	No response.
5	Request repetition, model, for example, "Try and say the whole sentence after me. Say, 'The man is crying because he hit his head.'"	Imitation. For example, "Hit head–crying"
6	Reinforce, model. For example, "Nice going! The man is crying because he hit his head."	

patient's spontaneous picture description in step 1. Referring to Table 16.1, the response to the step 3 "wh" cure, "hit head," was an elaboration of the original step 1 response, "crying."

In step 5 of the program an acceptable "imitation" was defined as an intelligible response containing one or more content words from both the spontaneous description (step 1) and the patient elaboration (step 3). An example of an acceptable imitation is also provided in Table 16.1. In this example the patient's step 5 response, "Hit head-crying" includes all content words produced in the patient's earlier spontaneous description (step 1) and his subsequent elaboration (step 3).

If an acceptable response was produced following a repetition of any step in the program, the subsequent step was administered and training continued. Alternately, if an unacceptable response was elicited following a repetition of a given step, then that portion of the training trial was terminated.

Recall that a training trial consisted of two "runs" or attempts to complete the six-step continuum. Thus, if the first run of a trial was terminated after a given step was unsuccessfully repeated, then the second run began by repeating step 1 for that *same* item. Alternately, if the second run of a training trial was terminated following an unsuccessful repetition, that training trial was terminated and another trial began for a *new* item.

As the training phase of the study progressed, Mike began to spontaneously produce increasingly more information in response to the training stimuli. These more elaborate responses were also prompted, chained, and modeled during each training trial until the training criterion was finally met. For example, Mike's spontaneous description of the sample item in Table 16.1 evolved from his initial "Crying" response to "Hit head-crying" to finally, "Ball hit head-crying-doctor see him."

Reliability. In order to assess the reliability of the clinician's scoring of Mike's responses, an independent observer rescored the three initial baseline sessions and the clinical probes administered when training criterion was reached for the two sets of training items. Interobserver agreement was calculated by comparing the clinician's scoring of these sessions with the observer's scores on a point-to-point basis for the number of content units produced in response to each stimulus item. The formula for computing interobserver agreement or reliability was:

$$\frac{\text{Reliability} = \text{agreements}}{\text{agreements \& disagreements} \times 100}$$

Agreement between the clinician and the independent observer for the number of content words produced in response to each item ranged from 80% to 97%. The average agreement across sessions was 88%. It can be inferred from these data that the clinician accurately scored Mike's responses.

RESULTS

Treatment

The results of Mike's treatment are presented in Figures 16.1, 16.2, and 16.3. Each figure displays performance on baseline and clinical probe tests administered throughout each phase of the study. Figure 16.1 depicts the number of responses which contained ≥ 5 content words for the two sets of training items. Examination of the top of Figure 16.1 reveals a stable rate of baseline responding to set 1 items. During the first three baseline sessions, a maximum of one response to the ten set 1 items contained five or more content words. Examination of the bottom of the Figure 16.1 also reveals a stable rate of baseline responding for set 2 items. Prior to intervention Mike typically produced one or two word telegraphic responses and elaborate responses. Those containing five or more content words were rarely produced.

Following the initiation of treatment for set 1 items (Figure 16.1), there was a gradual increase in the number of elaborate responses produced through the first ten probes. By the tenth probe the patient was consistently and spontaneously producing five or more content words in response to three of the set 1 items. After a rapid improvement in

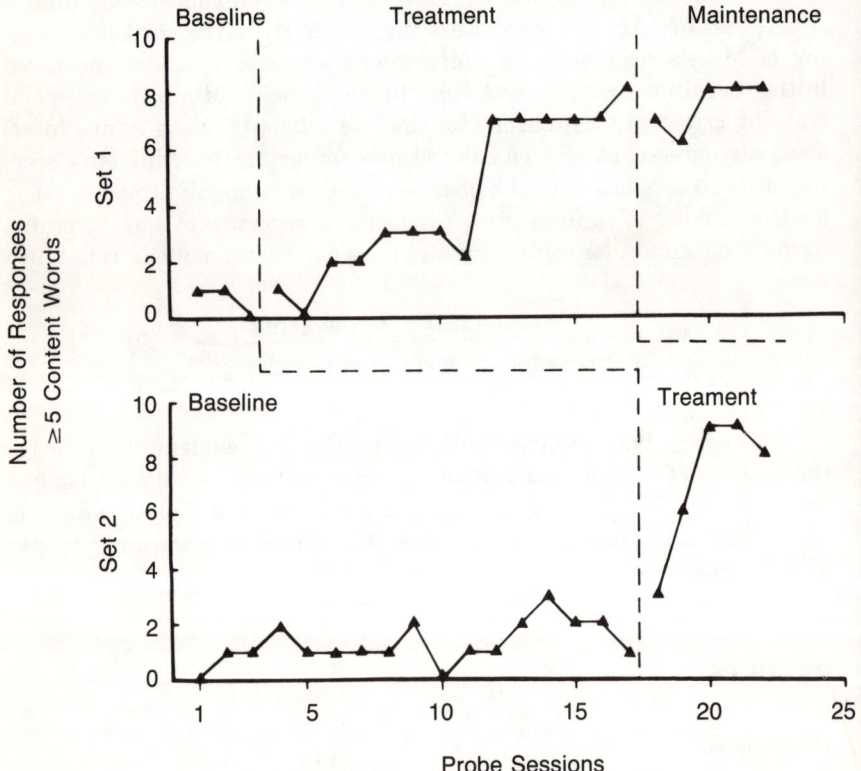

Figure 16.1 Number of responses having ≥5 content words for set 1 (top) and set 2 (bottom) training words during clinical probes. Baseline, Treatment, and Maintenance phrases are depicted.

Systematic Programming of Verbal Elaboration Skills   237

performance on the twelfth probe, Mike consistently produced ≥5 content words in response to 7 of the 10 set 1 items. Performance stabilized at this level until the seventeenth probe when eight of ten responses contained five or more content words. Since training criterion was met during this session, set 1 training was terminated, and treatment began on set 2 items during the next training session.

A total of 15 treatment sessions was needed to reach the training criterion. An examination of the "maintenance" phase (Figure 16.1) reveals that Mike continued to produce elaborate responses during follow-up probes (sessions 18–22) after set 1 training was terminated and treatment began for the second set of items.

As the lower portion of Figure 16.1 reveals, Mike's performance on set 2 items was stable prior to the initiation of treatment. He produced

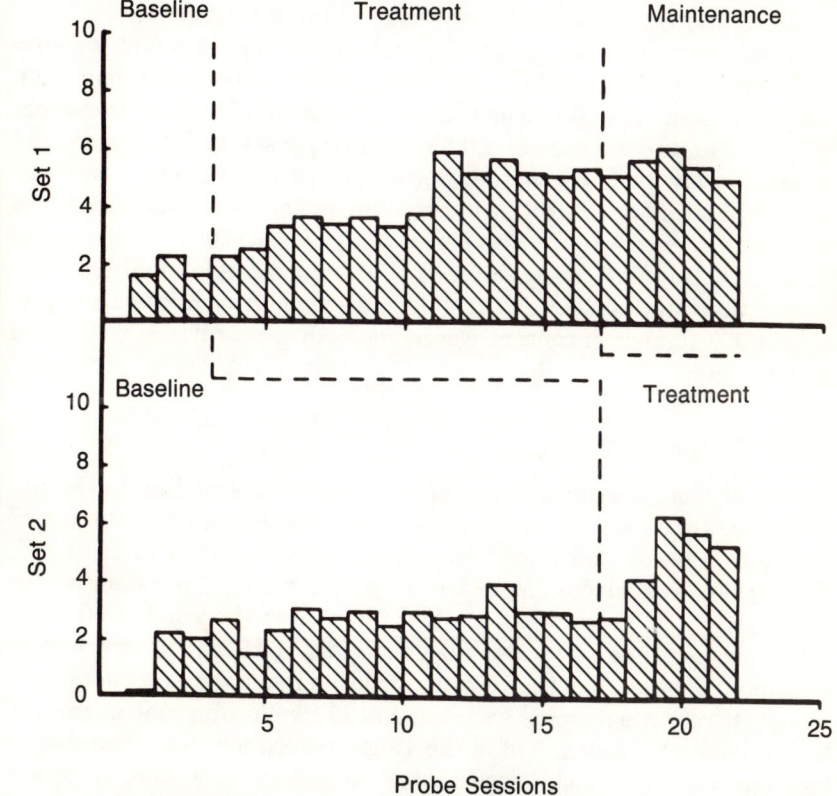

Figure 16.2 Mean number of content words produced for set 1 (top) and set 2 (bottom) training words during clinical probes. Baselin, Treatment, and Maintenance phases are depicted.

a maximum of three responses containing ≥5 content words on set 2 items during the first 17 probe sessions. Following the introduction of treatment (session 18), there was a marked and rapid increase in the number of elaborate responses produced to set 2 items. By the twentieth probe Mike produced five or more content words in response to 9 of the 10 training items. Since this performance exceeded the pre-established training criterion, training ceased for set 2 items and the study was completed. A total of six training sessions were conducted with set 2 stimuli.

The results of training for both sets of items revealed a considerable improvement over baseline performance. The program appeared to facilitate a marked increase in the amount of information supplied during spontaneous responses to the treatment stimuli. Significantly, improvement was apparent only after training was directly applied to the two sets of stimuli. These results support the conclusion that the experimental treatment program was effective for this patient.

Analysis of the mean number of content words produced in response to the two sets of stimuli in Figure 16.2 further supports the conclusion that treatment was effective. The mean number of content words per utterance was approximately 2.0 for set 1 responses, and it ranged from approximately 2.0 to 3.0 content words per response for set 2 items during the baseline phase. Following treatment, the mean number of content words per utterance was consistently above 5.0 for both sets of responses. The clinical significance of this increase is highlighted by noting that Mike essentially doubled the amount of information provided (i.e., number of content words) for both sets of items by the end of the study.

Generalization

The results of generalization of more elaborate responding to the ten untrained items are shown in Figure 16.3. Examination of the top of the figure reveals that a moderate degree of carry-over was exhibited. Whereas Mike produced one or zero responses having ≥5 content words during baseline, there was a gradual increase in the number of elaborate responses once treatment began on set 1 items. By the end of treatment on set 1, 6 of the 10 generalization items were produced with five or more content words each (session 17). Following continuation of training on set 2 items, half of the 10 generalization items had five or more content units each (session 22). Generalization of more elaborate responding was apparent for 50% of the untrained items.

The effect of the program on Mike's responses to the untrained items is also apparent by examining the data on the lower portion of Figure 16.3. It can be seen that the mean number of content words produced

Systematic Programming of Verbal Elaboration Skills 239

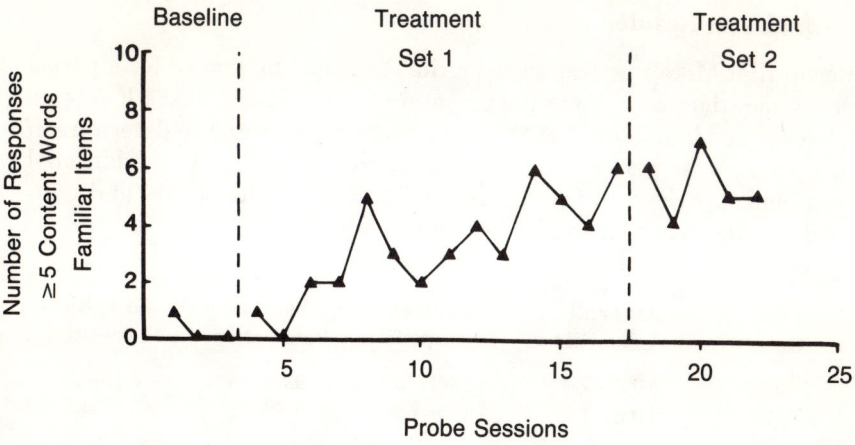

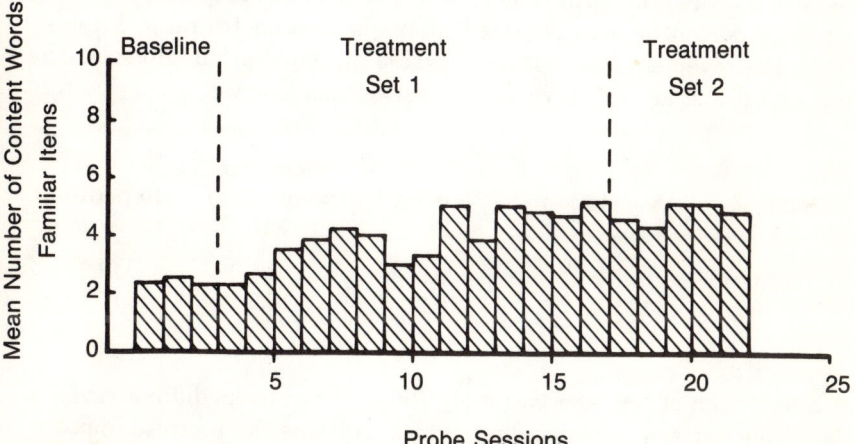

Figure 16.3 Generalization to untrained, familiar words. Number of responses having ≥5 content words produced are depicted in the bottom figure.

in response to untrained items improved from approximately 2.0 during baseline to nearly 5.0 at the termination of set 2 treatment. The amount of information (number of content words) produced to generalization items was significantly increased despite the fact that these items were never directly trained. It would appear, therefore, that the training program was both effective and efficient for facilitating response elaboration.

Formal Test Results

Recall that Mike's performance on the PICA had plateaued for a period of six months prior to his participation in this study. The PICA was, however, readministered at the completion of the study to determine if any change in performance was apparent following the additional treatment provided in this investigation. The results of pre- and poststudy performance on the PICA were as follows:

Date	Overall Percentile	Gestural Percentile	Verbal Percentile	Graphic Percentile
Pretest	10.65–46	13.38–66	9.58–44	7.75–53
Posttest	10.87–52	13.09–58	10.83–79	7.85–55

Examination of the pre- and poststudy test results reveals a slight overall improvement in posttest performance. This overall change appears to reflect improved performance on Verbal subtests where a score of 9.58/44 percentile was obtained before the study and a score of 10.83/79 percentile was obtained after elaboration training. Interestingly, improvement was apparent across all four Verbal subtests. The pre- and poststudy PICA Verbal scores were as follows:

Subtest	(Description) IV	(Naming) IX	(Sentence Completion) XII	(Repetition)
Prestudy	8.2	9.3	8.6	12.2
Poststudy	9.7	10.2	10.3	13.1

A comparison of pre- and poststudy PICA verbal tasks did not reveal a definitive pattern of responding, which explains the posttest improvement. However, there was an increase in accuracy and responsiveness evident on the posttest, particularly on PICA subtests I (description of function) and IX (sentence completion).

DISCUSSION

This multiple-baseline study provides convincing evidence that the treatment program facilitated an increase in Mike's response elaboration. In addition, a moderate degree of generalization of more elaborate responding was apparent for untrained, familiar items. Somewhat surprisingly, his performance on PICA verbal subtests also improved, despite the fact that he had plateaued on this measure prior to beginning elaboration training. Additional research is needed to determine if the elaboration training program would be equally effective for other aphasic patients.

The verbal elaboration training program examined in this study evolved from functional considerations which have been discussed in the recent aphasia literature. For example, one of the concerns expressed by Davis and Wilcox (1981) in their development of "PACE" was that didactic, clinician directed programs do not allow patients to share the burden of communication with their conversational partner. Clinicians often restrict patient communication to a narrow range of predetermined responses during highly structured didactic treatment. PACE is a purposeful departure from the unidirectional interaction of many traditional treatment approaches.

The verbal elaboration approach examined in this study also represents a significant departure from the clinician-controlled patient responding that typifies more directive treatment approaches. However, unlike PACE therapy where the clinician and patient alternately share the roles of sending and receiving messages, the *patient* is purposefully given the primary burden of communication in the present approach. That is, with verbal elaboration training the patient actually directs the course of treatment, because his spontaneous descriptions and elaborations are the primary focus of treatment. Mike's clinician, for example, did not preselect or restrict his responses, and clinician elaborations were kept to a minimum. In a sense, the clinician acted as a therapeutic navigator by ensuring that the patient was on proper course, but the patient himself mapped out the direction of elaboration training. This aspect of the program is similar to the philosophy underlying a conversational prompting technique described by McCrae-Cochrane and Milton (1984).

Contrary to our initial concern, the elaboration program did not appear to interfere seriously with interactive aspects of communication. This may, in part, reflect the fact that normal individuals often seek clarification and elaboration from aphasic individuals during everyday interactions. Another factor that may have contributed to maintaining an active exchange of information relates to the treatment techniques themselves. Specifically, the prompting and reinforcing of novel, appropriate responses that were not directly depicted in treatment stimuli resulted in production of a diverse vocabulary and a variety of themes. This aspect of treatment helped to keep the approach from being overly repetitive, and it kept the interaction bidirectional. Perhaps, as Chapey's (1981) discussion of divergent semantic approach suggests, programs that "loosen" patient response requirements during treatment may result in creative, flexible language use that more closely approximates naturalistic communication.

As previously noted, the limited data provided by this patient does not permit conclusions regarding the usefulness of elaboration training with other aphasic individuals. Additional research is being conducted to examine the generality of this treatment approach. Despite its limitations, however, this clinical investigation highlights several important aspects of clinical intervention that deserve further mention.

One noteworthy aspect of the present study is that it demonstrates the importance of obtaining clinical data from actual treatment tasks. Formal test data alone are often insufficient for making routine clinical decisions, and ongoing clinical data can be used to enhance and supplement formal test results. It is not, for example, unusual for there to be a poor correlation between clinical treatment data and the results of standard aphasia assessments. Although it was not the case in the present study, patients frequently evidence good progress on treatment tasks that is not reflected in test results. Such discrepancies may effect dismissal and other important clinical decisions. As this study demonstrates, judicious use of clinical treatment data is often invaluable for determining the exact nature and pattern of change over time. By design, the global nature of aphasia tests do not provide the ongoing information needed to make adjustments in clinical tasks or treatment direction. In many instances standardized testing is necessary, but it is not a sufficient means of assessing aphasic individuals and making clinical management decisions.

Treatment approaches that emphasize the collection of ongoing clinical data are, of course, only as good as the clinicians who employ them. Clinical data do not remove the decision-making process from the clinician. Rather, the systematic collection of clinical data provides the clinician with a judgment aid that may contribute valuable information to the decision-making process. There are a number of data-based treatment approaches presently available to assist the clinician in evaluating treatment effectiveness. For example, numerous experimental designs, such as the multiple baseline design used in this study, can be employed with minimal disruption of normal clinical routine (McReynolds & Kearns, 1983). Incorporation of these and similar design strategies into our clinical repertoire may provide a more principled and objective means of treating aphasic individuals.

ACKNOWLEDGEMENT

The writing of this manuscript was supported in part by Veterans Administration Medical Research Funds. The helpful suggestions of Nina N. Simmons are also greatly appreciated.

REFERENCES

Chapey, R. (1981). Divergent semantic intervention. In R. Chapey (Ed.), *Language intervention strategies in adult aphasia*. Baltimore: Williams & Wilkins.

Davis, G.A., & Wilcox, M.J. (1981). Incorporating parameters of natural conversation in aphasia treatment. In R. Chapey (Ed.), *Language intervention strategies in adult aphasia*. Baltimore: Williams & Wilkins.

Fokes, J. (1976). *Fokes Sentence Builder*. New York: Teaching Resources.

Hart, B. (1981). Pragmatics: How language is used. *Analysis and Intervention in Developmental Disabilities, 1*, 299–313.

Hart, B., & Risley, T.R. (1974). Using preschool materials to modify the language of disadvantaged children. *Journal of Applied Behavior Analysis, 7*(2), 243–256.

Holland, A.D. (1977). Some practical considerations in aphasia rehabilitation. In M. Sullivan and M.S. Kommers (Eds.), *Rationale for adult aphasia therapy*. Omaha: University of Nebraska Medical Center Print Shop.

McCrae-Cochran R., & Milton, S.B. (1984). Conversational prompting: A sentence building technique for severe aphasia. *Journal of Neurological Communication Disorders, 1*, 4–23.

McReynolds, L.V., & Kearns, K.P. (1983). *Single-subject experimental designs in communication disorders*. Austin, TX: PRO-ED.

Porch, B.E. (1967). *Porch Index of Communicative Ability* (Vol. 2). Palo Alto, CA: Consulting Psychologists Press.

Skelly, M. (1979). *Amer-Ind gestural code bases on universal American Indian hand talk*. New York: Elsevier.

Stokes, T.F., & Baer, D.M. (1977). An implicit technology of generalization. *Journal of Applied Behavior Analysis 10*, 349–367.

APPENDIX A: Distribution of Stimulus Items

I. Set I Training Items

1. Cutting
2. Combing
3. Hitting
4. Catching
5. Crying
6. Swimming
7. Eating
8. Shooting
9. Dancing
10. Kicking

II. Set II Training Items

1. Ringing
2. Drawing
3. Punching
4. Cutting
5. Stirring
6. Slipping
7. Fishing
8. Calling
9. Swinging
10. Laughing

III. Generalization Items—Previous Exposure

1. Throwing
2. Sweeping
3. Hammering
4. Giving
5. Reading
6. Writing
7. Washing
8. Pouring
9. Running
10. Singing

CHAPTER 17

Computers and Caring

Russell H. Mills and Pamela C. Hoffer

> The computer revolution has had an impact upon the field of speech-language-pathology. Mills and Hoffer describe how microcomputers were used to augment clinicians' efforts in the treatment of language and cognitive deficits of two clients. They offer their insights on the traditional and nontraditional applications of microcomputers in treatment. The former involved using the technology to provide massed practice in auditory and reading comprehension for an aphasic client. The latter entailed teaching a head-injured client to use the word processor and other features of the computer to compensate for his cognitive deficits.
>
> 1. Describe the microcomputer programs used with Mills and Hoffer's aphasic client. What were the advantages and disadvantages of using these programs? Describe the programs used with their head-injured patient. How did microcomputer treatment assist him at different stages of his recovery? How did each client's training differ?
> 2. The authors point out that microcomputer instruction comprised a small portion of their clients' treatment. Summarize their philosophy with respect to the roles of the microcomputer and clinician in the total treatment process. Do you think computers are effective treatment tools? why or why not?

INTRODUCTION

This chapter describes how microcomputer technology was employed in the management of two patients. The first is Chuck, a 39-year-old male, who exhibited a severe aphasia and apraxia secondary to a left hemisphere CVA. The second, Steve, is a 26-year-old male who exhibited a variety of linguistic and nonlinguistic dysfunctions secondary to brain injury suffered in a motor vehicle accident. Chuck's report details the traditional use of specific software to help rebuild the basic linguistic skills of auditory and reading comprehension. Our report of Steve's treatment describes how the computer was utilized nontraditionally to promote communication when the patient's basic language skills remained intact but other cognitive deficits (e.g., memory) persisted.

The reader should recognize that in neither case was treatment relegated solely to the microcomputer. At the time Chuck and Steve first began treatment there was a limited array of software and peripheral devices available. While the number of these devices has increased over the last four years, microcomputerized treatment has not replaced traditional methodologies. Its proper role, however, is as a powerful clinical tool that can significantly augment the services provided by the clinician. Successful utilization of this technology requires that the clinician recognize both its strengths and limitations.

THE CASE: CHUCK

Background Information and Medical History

Chuck was a 39-year-old computer programming supervisor. He had been married for 12 years and had two children. In September 3, 1979, he traveled to Indiana for a baseball game. That evening he became ill and retired early. When he awoke in the morning, he was unable to speak. He was taken successively to two area hospitals, but his condition deteriorated throughout the day. Chuck was transferred to a major university medical center where cerebral angiography revealed a complete occlusion of the left internal carotid artery. The next day he exhibited a dense global aphasia, verbal apraxia, right hemiparesis, and probable right homonymous hemianopsia. He remained in the hospital until November 16, 1979, during which time he received speech and language treatment and physical and occupational therapies. Although Chuck's aphasic deficits improved slightly during his hospital course, he continued to reflect severe limitations in all language modalities at discharge. For example, he was inconsistent in his ability to follow single commands, repeat short phrases, point to single words, and write his name. The general feeling was that he had reached maximum recovery. After discharge Chuck received speech and language treatment in his home once a week. The family requested more intensive treatment but the request was denied on the basis that Chuck was not changing significantly. The family ultimately sought treatment at the Ann Arbor Veterans Administration Medical Center. Chuck began treatment there in January 1981 at six months postonset.

Speech and Language Evaluation

Chuck's Overall and modality mean scores and percentile rankings on the *Porch Index of Communication Ability* (PICA) (Porch, 1967) are shown in Table 17.1. His 34th percentile Overall ranking reflects the severity of his impairment. On the Auditory Comprehension subtests of the PICA he could point to common objects when their names were spoken by the examiner with 70% accuracy but dropped to 20% success when their functions were given. *Token Test* results (Spreen & Benton, 1969) placed Chuck at the 18th percentile in a normative group of adult subjects. He could retain four digits forward and two digits backward. In most tests auditory comprehension was deleteriously influenced by reduced auditory memory span.

TABLE 17.1
PICA Results Throughout Chuck's Treatment Program

DATE	OVERALL	GESTURAL	VERBAL	GRAPHIC
JAN '81	8.82 (34)*	11.20 (29)	6.18 (31)	7.40 (48)
JAN '82	10.49 (49)	12.45 (45)	8.57 (40)	9.30 (69)
JAN '83	11.59 (62)	12.78 (51)	10.38 (47)	9.70 (72)
AUG '84	11.81 (65)	13.56 (70)	10.91 (49)	10.08 (74)
CHANGE	+31%ILE	+41%ILE	+18%ILE	+26%ILE

*(nn) = Percentile based on left hemisphere norms

Chuck's reading was similarly impaired. On the visual matching subtests of the *Minnesota Test for Differential Diagnosis of Aphasia* (MTDDA) (Schuell, 1965) he matched geometric forms correctly but matched only 60% of the letters presented. These results indicated the presence of a visual perceptual processing disturbance exclusive of his reading comprehension difficulties. In PICA reading subtests V and VII, 55% of his responses were correct but incomplete. In no instance did he correctly appreciate the prepositions present in the written stimuli (e.g., Put this card to the *left* of the cigarettes). Performance on the *Reading*

Comprehension Battery for Aphasia (RCBA) (LaPointe & Horner, 1979) was also severely restricted. Chuck responded at a 60% success rate for the first three subtests requiring the comprehension of single words. He produced only one correct response in the functional reading subtest, and then the RCBA was discontinued.

Verbal expression was severely limited. Chuck could repeat only three of ten PICA object names. Responses in sentence completion, naming, or sentence formulation tasks were inaccurate. In our apraxia battery Chuck's diadochokinetic rates for /p/ and /t/ were slightly below normal limits; he was unable to produce /k/, or a single /p/-/t/-/k/ combination. He imitated less than 10% of the single words presented. He had much less difficulty producing nonverbal oral movements, and it was concluded that his severe limitation in verbal responding was due, to a significant degree, to the presence of a severe verbal apraxia.

Chuck's written responses were nonfunctional. He could copy geometric forms and a few words but did not write any names of pictures, his name, serial numbers, or spell to dictation.

Microcomputer Task Selection

The global nature of Chuck's aphasia warranted a careful, wide-ranging plan of care. We recognized that the severity of his impairments at 6 months postonset suggested his potential was limited, but neither he nor his family accepted these limitations. The tasks on which he had difficulty in formal testing (e.g., pointing to objects named; pointing to objects described by function; reading; matching letters) could be administered by microcomputer. Moreover, Chuck had been a computer programmer, and we felt he might be particularly enthusiastic about computerized treatment. Finally, we believed that computerized treatment might facilitate rehabilitation.

We selected an Apple II+ system for Chuck's treatment, but we did not know how well he would use this system, and that he would ultimately help us develop some of our own programs over the next four years. During this time, Chuck received many forms of treatment: individual, group, home based, telecommunicology (Fitch & Cross, 1983), clinical-based and home-based computerized treatment. When our microcomputer offered a distinct advantage, we used it (e.g., auditory comprehension, reading, math), but where hardware or software limitations existed, other methods were employed. Chuck made slow, steady progress in all of his therapeutic endeavors. This chapter, however, only describes the ways in which the microcomputer was used to improve his auditory comprehension and reading skills.

Auditory Comprehension Training. Results of Chuck's initial evaluation suggested his auditory processing was impaired because of several factors. He had increasing difficulty as message length and rate of speech increased. Inclusion of verbs and prepositions increased semantic/syntactic complexity and memory load, and further impaired his comprehension. Some of these problems could be addressed systematically in an auditory comprehension program entitled *Word Recognition Programs* (Word Rec) (Brain-Link Software). The Word Rec programs produce digitized speech through a device called the Mountain Computer Supertalker SD-200. The speech, digitized at a rate of 4,000 samples per second, results in a message that sounds human and is highly intelligible.

Chuck received concentrated training with three of six available programs, Word Rec I, II, and III. All were similar in their manner of execution. They presented plates of four line drawings of common objects as visual stimuli on the monitor screen. In Word Rec I the computer directed Chuck to find a single object whose name was produced by the speech digitizer. In Word Rec II a sequence of two, and in Word Rec III a sequence of three names was given. Chuck responded by pressing a key on the keyboard. A press of the "return" key provided him with a repeat of the stimulus. The Word Rec programs also allowed the clinician to manipulate parameters such as rate of speech and response input method. Text prompting was provided on the monitor screen, and a variety of reinforcers followed each response. Data collection/analysis routines recorded correct and incorrect responses, response times in milliseconds, and calculated mean percent for correct and incorrect responses, mean response times, and standard deviations.

In 1983 two more auditory comprehension programs from Brainlink software were added to Chuck's program. The first, *Function Recognition*, provides training in the comprehension of spoken verbs and verb sequences. A second, *Preposition Recognition*, provides training in the comprehension of spoken prepositions and preposition sequences. These programs operate similarly to the Word Rec programs.

Of his six hours of weekly treatment, approximately one fourth was devoted to microcomputer training. Chuck worked on the Word Rec, Function Rec, and Prep Rec programs at different times in the course of his treatment. Following their introduction he practiced on each program until a criterion level of 90% correct responding across three consecutive trials with less than four stimulus repeats per 20 items was achieved. He then discontinued regular practice at the level of difficulty, but periodic probes continued to be administered.

Reading Comprehension Training. Chuck's reading performance during his initial evaluation indicated both visual perceptual and reading comprehension disturbances. Computerized reading comprehension training began with visual perceptual tasks. Treatment then proceeded using reading comprehension tasks of increasing difficulty maintaining the 90% criterion. The major reading comprehension programs employed with Chuck and the order in which they were administered are given in Table 17.4. As in his auditory comprehension training, all of the programs were not available when Chuck entered the program.

The first program introduced was the *Preschool I.Q. Builder* by EduWare. In this program, single letters were presented on the screen. Chuck's task was to press the corresponding letter on the keyboard. Feedback was provided in the form of a "beep" (correct) or a "buzz" (incorrect). Another program, *Shell Games* (Apple Computer), provided the framework for developing several perceptual and reading comprehension tasks. A matching format was used first in which one of ten items from column A had to be matched to the correct item in column B using the keyboard letter and number selections. The first task required the matching of identical column A and B words of four letters or less. Task difficulty was increased by adding more visually confusing words to a list. Later versions required the matching words of seven to nine letters. Matching was also employed in a second program with a different format, *Square Pairs* (Scholastic), which presented stimuli in a concentration game. This program was employed to work on synonyms, antonyms, noun-verb (e.g., ball-bounce), and adjective-noun (e.g., red-apple) associations.

As Chuck's reading comprehension improved, the multiple choice and true and false portions of *Shell Games* provided him more complex reading exercises and promoted the comprehension of phrase, sentence, and paragraph length materials. In all of these exercises Chuck had only to select his choice from the stimuli presented on the monitor screen. This recognition format was selected because early in treat-

TABLE 17.2
Chuck's Performance in Microcomputer Auditory Comprehension Tasks

Date	Word Rec I	Word Rec II	Word Rec III	Function Rec	Prep Rec
Jan '81	91.6% (4)*	58.0% (8)	10.0% (2)	---- ---	---- ---
May '81	100.0% (0)	91.6% (1)	41.6% (33)	---- ---	---- ---
Jan '82	100.0% (0)	100.0% (0)	83.0% (8)	---- ---	---- ---
Jan '83	100.0% (0)	91.6% (0)	78.0% (6)	46.6% (4)	---- ---
Jan '84	93.3% (0)	95.0% (1)	83.3% (5)	60.0% (6)	35.0% (9)
Mar '84	100.0% (0)	100.0% (2)	75.0% (4)	50.0% (8)	78.0% (3)
Aug '84	100.0% (0)	95.0% (1)	80.0% (4)	93.3% (3)	83.3% (0)

* = Number of stimulus repeats employed during a 20 item trial

ment Chuck's spelling ability precluded his responding otherwise. In later stages of his treatment the *Game Show* and *Tic Tac Show* programs (Advanced Ideas) were introduced and Chuck was able to type his responses. These treatment sequences were entertaining and of interest to Chuck. Typically, Chuck was presented with a short reading passage on the screen and then asked to type the answers to questions regarding the content of the passage. In later exercises the computer program was combined with traditional reading materials. For example, Chuck was given a short newspaper article, an advertisement, or a section of a map to read. Following the reading of these materials, the computer was programmed to test his comprehension and memory of the materials.

Results

Auditory Comprehension. Table 17.2 provides selected data for Chuck's performance on the Word Rec programs. Values reflect a mean of three 20-item trials of a program. In January of 1981 when he began treatment, Chuck met criterion on the Word Rec I program (91.6%). This high level of performance was predicted based on the results of his initial evaluation. In the Word Rec II and III programs he had much greater difficulty. Because increased length of the message sequence appeared to contribute to Chuck's poorer performance on programs II and III, a response contingent delay was employed in administering these programs. The rate of speech was reduced one step following an error and increased one step following a correct response. The computer was capable of generating four rates of computerized speech production. The most rapid approximated normal speech, while the slowest averaged 50 words per minute. By May of 1981 Chuck made no errors on Word Rec I, performed at the 90% criterion on Word Rec II, but was still having problems with Word Rec III. After a year in the program (January of 1982), Chuck regularly met criterion for Word Rec level I and II, and level III scores had doubled to 83% correct but with 8 repeats in 20 trials. At this point practice on Word Rec I and II was terminated. Chuck continued to work on Level III, but he was unable to reach 90% success.

Chuck began the Function Rec verb program in January, 1983. Table 17.2 shows that he made steady improvement on this program and by August of 1984 reached criterion level. Chuck is currently working on the second level of Function Rec involving two-verb stimuli. So far his highest level of performance has been 75% correct. The computer data and Chuck's continued difficulty on Subtest VI of the PICA indicate that the comprehension of verbs is a difficult task for Chuck, whether presented by computer or the clinician.

In January 1984 the Preposition Rec program was introduced. His beginning level of performance was 35% correct. With repeated practice, use of the response contingent delay, and repeat features, his August 1984 performance on this program had reached 83% correct. He has been given trial practice on a second level Preposition Rec Program, but scores remain unstable, ranging from 65% to 80% correct.

Response Latency. Response Latency (RT) data provided a second measure of Chuck's auditory comprehension performance. RT data presented in Table 17.3 indicate that when Chuck began treatment, his mean RTs for the Word Rec programs were 9.782, 21.541, and 26.170 seconds for Levels I, II, and III, respectively. Mean RTs for normal adults range from approximately one to three seconds for the same tasks. Table 17.3 shows that Chuck reduced his mean latency time in all Word Rec Programs with treatment. Similar processing time reductions for the Function Rec and Preposition Rec programs were also noted. More important, his family reported that reduced response latencies have carried over into functional communication situations and increased his effectiveness.

TABLE 17.3
Change in Mean Response Times (Seconds) of Correct Responses in Three Auditory Comprehension Tasks

Date	Word Rec I	Word Rec II	Word Rec III	Function Rec	Prep Rec I
Jan '81	9.782	21.541	16.170	-----	-----
Jan '83'	2.970	11.534	19.060	8.527	-----
Jan '84	3.125	7.090	10.373	6.340	7.255
Dec '84	2.850	6.955	9.677	5.656	3.334
CHANGE	−6.932	−14.586	−6.493	−2.871	−3.921

Reading Comprehension. Table 17.4 provides a summary of Chuck's scores on the reading comprehension programs. Because the programs were introduced at different times, the midway measures reflect a performance level halfway between baseline and criterion or his highest level of performance.

Results indicate that at the beginning of treatment Chuck had difficulty matching single letters, four-letter, and nine-letter words. Computer treatment resulted in rapid and significant improvement in matching. Chuck reached criterion on these three programs in nine weeks and continues to perform flawlessly when periodically retested. Generalization to noncomputerized tasks was demonstrated when he elevated his score on the Matching Letters subtest of the MTDDA to 100% following completion of these three programs.

TABLE 17.4
Change in Performance in Computerized
Reading Comprehension Tasks

TASK	PROGRAM	EARLY	MIDWAY	FINAL
Single Letter Match	Preschool I.Q.	76%	82%	100%
Four Letter Word Match	Shell Games	55%	75%	100%
Nine Letter Word Match	Shell Games	25%	45%	92%
Noun-Verb Match	Shell Games	25%	65%	83%
Noun-Verb Memory Match	Square Pairs	10%	63%	87%
Sentence Comp. (True/False)	Shell Games	45%	75%	86%
News Article Comprehension (Recognition Task)	Game Show Tic-Tac-Show	10%	30%	56%
News Article Comprehension (Recall Task)	Game Show Tic-Tac-Show	10%	35%	30%

Chuck has shown equally significant gains on programs that require responses based on meaning. Performance in the noun-verb, noun-pronoun and adjective-noun matching programs has improved. Representative improvement is shown in Table 17.4 for the "Noun-Verb Match" task. While he fell slightly short of criterion on this task (83%) on his final test, he missed only low frequency word combinations. He continues to work on these matching programs in which the words are frequently changed. When the noun-verb task was placed in *Square Pairs* format taxing short-term and recent memory, early performance was even more impaired than in the task that was not memory weighted. However, performance has steadily improved to the point that Chuck frequently nears or meets criterion in this task as well.

The reading tasks provided by the *Game Show* and *Tic Tac Show* programs are most similar to functional reading requirements. Table 17.4 shows that Chuck improved to 56% correct on the tasks that required recognition responses, but it should be pointed out that he rarely exceeded 35% on tasks where he was required to recall his response choice. The assessment of recall performance is complicated by the requirement to spell the response correctly, and Chuck continued to exhibit a severe spelling disorder. This deficit has been addressed by computer and traditional techniques several times in the treatment setting, but Chuck's spelling ability has not shown improvement to functional levels.

Summary of Chuck's Case Study

The PICA results presented in Table 17.1 reflect an improvement in Chuck's Overall language performance in all modalities over the course of all treatment. Other measures (RCBA), *Token Test,* Digit Span) reflected similar changes. Because of the long-term nature of Chuck's treatment and the multifaceted program employed, it is difficult to determine to what extent computerized treatment contributed to these gains.

Several points about Chuck's treatment and progress can be made. First, whatever factors are operating, Chuck improved significantly following dismissal from treatment in 1981. His improvement over a four year period indicates that significant change is possible in chronic aphasia. Second, Chuck's auditory comprehension of nouns, verbs, and prepositions, understanding of conversational speech, and retention of word sequences have improved, and he has shown similar gains in reading comprehension. Although we cannot be certain whether the skills learned on the computer resulted in gains on the PICA, *Token Test,* MTDDA, and RCBA, specific areas of greatest improvement were those which were emphasized in the computer training program. Most important, improvement in functional communication was observed by his clinicians, friends, wife, and children. We are sufficiently convinced of the value of the computer training for Chuck and its potential use in the clinic and in the home for other aphasic patients.

THE CASE: STEVE

Background Information and Medical History

Steve is a 26-year-old, right handed man who suffered severe closed-head injuries in a motor vehicle accident. He is a graduate of West Point in engineering with a history of academic and athletic achievement. Steve is married to Laura and has a son, Scott, who was 3½ years old at the time of his father's injury.

On November 11, 1982, Steve, in a coma, was admitted to a hospital near the accident. He remained comatose for several weeks and gradually progressed from level four to eight on the Glasgow Coma Scale (Teasdale & Jennett, 1974). A CT scan showed a left thalamic hemorrhage, with damage to the adjacent internal capsule, and swelling of the left lateral ventricle. He was transferred to the Ann Arbor VA Medical Center at two and one half months postonset (MPO). He was intubated and fed through a nasogastric tube. At this time his rating on the Glasgow scale was 10. Steve demonstrated some spontaneous movement, but his response to sensory stimuli, including deep pain, was poor. He appeared mildly aware of activity around him, roused when his name was called, and followed objects with his gaze. He was able to follow simple commands with gaze changes. He did not, however, initiate any activity or attempt to communicate.

Speech and Language Evaluation

Steve was a challenge to evaluate. Some of the medical staff concluded he was in a persistent vegetative state. He was mute and had little voluntary tongue or facial movement, and no voluntary phonation or breath control. The key difficulty in testing him was that his response latencies were extremely slow (often 15 seconds to begin a thumb signal). His cognitive abilities were often perceived incorrectly, because he could not give his responses quickly enough. In the same day that a note appeared in his chart describing him as being in a "persistent vegetative state," he demonstrated that he could (a) read simple commands, (b) understand spoken language that was syntactically straightfoward, and (c) answer questions using an up/down thumb movement to indicate yes or no.

Assessing Steve's intellectual and communicative abilities was a long-term process. Tests administered between two and four months postonset included all or parts of the following: the *Boston Diagnostic Aphasia Examination* (BDAE) (Goodglass & Kaplan, 1972); the *Peabody Picture Vocabulary Test* (PPVT) (Dunn & Dunn, 1981); the *Reading Comprehension Battery for Aphasia* (RCBA) (LaPointe & Horner, 1979); and the *Motor Free Visual Perception Test* (MFVPT) (Colarusso & Hammill, 1972). Substantial informal testing and/or observations were also carried out in this time.

Amnestic Deficits. Steve had severe retrograde and anterograde amnesia. He could not remember daily events until eight months after his insult. Short-term memory for both visual input (block span: 5 forward and 5 backward) and auditory input (digit span: 6 forward and 3 backward) was better than his memory for events, but was reduced from premorbid levels.

Comprehension. Steve's auditory and reading comprehension were relatively intact, but he had difficulty retaining information in both modalities. Initial testing of auditory comprehension indicated he could respond correctly to BDAE yes/no questions (e.g., Will a board sink in water?) with his thumb signal, but he scored only 58% correct on the BDAE comprehension subtest requiring retention of paragraph-length material. Although Steve was extremely slow to respond, he scored 80% correct on reading comprehension of sentences on the BDAE and 90% correct on the functional reading subtest of the RCBA. The PPVT test of receptive vocabulary yielded an IQ equivalent of 89. Assessment of reading comprehension was complicated by visual perceptual problems. On a test of visual perception he made 11 errors in 36 items, and evidenced particular difficulty with visual closure and figure ground relationships. However, four months later Steve made no errors. Ophthamological testing revealed convergence and scanning problems, and Steve was fitted with a prism lens to compensate for these difficulties during reading.

Speech and Language. Steve exhibited a severe spastic dysarthria. He did not achieve voluntary voicing until five months post-injury at which time he appeared to demonstrate a laryngeal-respiratory apraxia. He gradually became able to perform both vegetative and speech-related oral-motor tasks voluntarily, but movements remained extremely slow. He typically took 90 minutes to finish a meal with assistance from the staff.

Steve demonstrated good confrontation and responsive naming on the BDAE by mouthing words, but performance was below his previous academic achievement. Verbal fluency, as assessed by the animal-naming subtest of the BDAE, was also depressed. This deficit, however, seemed broader than a word-finding problem, perhaps reflecting reduction in ideational fluency. As Steve became more verbal, his language seemed elliptical, limited in content, and structurally awkward. These problems appeared related to a cognitive, memory, and organizational impairment, not an aphasic difficulty.

Writing. Initially, Steve's writing was severely limited by motor control, visual perceptual, and spelling impairments. By four months postonset, however, he regained enough spelling ability to use the Canon handheld typewriter or a Magic Slate. Generally, his messages were incomplete and somewhat confused. Despite the fact he could communicate by writing and laborious speaking, Steve did not initiate any communication for months. He remained silent, responding only to the communicative initiatives of those around him.

TREATMENT

Steve's treatment had three phases: an *inpatient phase,* a *dependent outpatient phase,* and an *independent outpatient phase.* The computer was introduced in the first, expanded in the second, and became central in the third phase, when he was loaned a microcomputer system for home use. The system employed throughout Steve's rehabilitation program was the Apple II+ by Apple Computer. It consisted of an Apple II+ 48k CPU, Zenith color monitor, Epson MX-80 printer, and joystick.

Phase I: Inpatient Treatment (2½ to 6 MPO)

Early in his inpatient treatment Steve was basically disconnected from others and himself, a condition resulting from his severe amnesia for past and current events. This deficit was compounded by his inability to vocalize or initiate the use of an augmentative system, and by his physical dependency. Early treatment concentrated on helping Steve feel safe, supported, and understood. We provided him with information about his present condition and his past history. The staff kept a running journal of the day's events and reviewed his photograph albums and personal address book with him. A communication board was developed to enhance his nonvocal communication. During this time we did not demand that he initiate communication, but provided him communication opportunities in which he could respond to questions by use of a thumb signal.

Humor was an important aspect of early treatment. Jokes were a useful means of promoting cognitive flexibility and abstract thinking. They also reinforced Steve to listen and remain attentive. As Steve became able to express himself with the Canon Communicator, we realized that we had "primed the pump" and that he possessed his own dry wit.

In the later stages of inpatient treatment, Steve was introduced to the microcomputer. Programs selected required him to sustain attention, decrease reaction time, make decisions, and perform visual memory and visual scanning tasks. (See Appendix A for the list of programs used and their target goals.) The first programs required single keypress responses. One, *React* from the *Cog Rehab Programs* package, measured the time required to press a key when a number was displayed at a location on the monitor screen. A second, *Search,* trained visual scanning by requiring a target shape be located in an array of many shapes. Another, *Sink the Ship,* required Steve with a single key press to drop a "bomb" from a plane on the deck of a ship that was moving in the opposite direction. Task difficulty was increased by varying the velocity of the plane and ship. This program proved to be useful in improving Steve's attention and his time-estimation judgments.

A programmed maze exercise operated with a joystick was introduced to help Steve sustain attention. His task was to move through the maze as rapidly as possible. Contacts with the walls of the maze constituted errors. Steve's progress was reflected by reduction in error scores and time to complete the maze program. Representative data are: 8 MPO: 115″, 76 errors; 12 MPO: 83″, 28 errors; 15 MPO: 35″, 22 errors; 19 MPO: 33″, 10 errors. Other programs involving reading comprehension and general information practice were introduced at the end of the inpatient period. We let Steve's interest dictate which programs were used. His response to the computer was enthusiastic. Although he had enjoyed his more traditional treatment sessions, he conveyed overt excitement in response to the computer as he found something that he could *do* successfully, not just say.

Inpatient treatment also focused on ameliorating his spastic dysarthia and improving speech intelligibility. Steve's occasional involuntary groaning on effort during physical therapy was used as a scaffold on which to rebuild voluntary voicing. He was also fitted with a palatal lift to compensate for excessive nasal emission, and articulation treatment was provided to help him overcome the severe distortions of vowels and consonants resulting from his spastic dysarthria.

Phase II: Dependent Outpatient (7 to 12 MPO)

In Phase II we encouraged Steve to expand his repertoire of communication partners and situations. He and his family also needed emotional support after he returned home. This was a stressful time. His family wanted him at home, but he was dependent on them for most of his needs. He remained severely dysarthric, usually unintelligible to his four-year-old son, and rarely initiated conversation. He was often depressed and felt that he was "empty," and "worthless," without anything meaningful to do. Treatment during this period included expanding the role of the computer, counseling Steve individually and with his wife, and providing dysarthria treatment focused on improving his intelligibility so his son could better understand him.

Computer Based Therapy. The computer now became an important part of Steve's rehabilitation in two ways. First, it allowed him to work independently on his cognitive and memory deficits. He used a speed-reading program *Compu-Read* and various reading comprehension programs that tested his ability to determine the main idea, note detail, and make inferences *(Understanding Sentences, Understanding Stories,* and *Micro Read).* Low level math drills *(Alien Addition, Minus Mission,* and *Meteor Multiplication)* were useful in promoting faster decision making, while SAT preparation programs *(SAT* and *SAT English)* allowed him to review the logical operations involved in higher level math and algebra skills. Of benefit to Steve's self-esteem was the fact that as he reviewed math and reading skills, he discovered abilities that remained relatively intact and improved deficit areas.

Second, and perhaps more important, the computer had substantial psychotherapeutic value. Steve learned to use the *Bank Street Writer* word processor to write letters to family and friends. In the process he discovered for himself and exhibited to others that much of his intelligence, wit, and personality had remained. Using the word processor, he could bypass his handwriting difficulties, but it still took him two hours to draft a one page letter. His difficulties in creating text on the word processor did not result from motoric difficulties, but from his ideational impairments and inability to initiate a task. When he first began to use the word processor, he was not sure that he could think of anything to write. However, when the computer printed what he had labored over, he realized that he did have something to say. The word processor allowed him to read what he had written, to correct mistakes, and to alter sentences. Furthermore, it allowed him to produce material that did not display his deficits. This accomplishment was invaluable in reinforcing his self-esteem and would not have been possible without the computer. The difference in his handwritten letters and those composed on the word processor was striking. The former were usually lacking in information, repetitive, and consisted of rambling comments about how long it took him to write the last sentence. Letters composed on the word processor were full of information about what he was doing and thinking and reflected a witty, conversational style.

Steve learned to use the word processor over a period of several months. He needed much structure and prompting. In his first attempt to answer a letter, he could not formulate a response. However, when he read individual sentences of his friends' letters he generated an appropriate reply to each. His first letter was six sentences long and took him an hour to compose. While he remains slow in writing letters, he works independently and is adept at communicating his feelings and ideas with the word processor (See Appendix 8 for longitudinal examples of his writing on the word processor.)

The word processor was also used to increase ideational fluency. One technique encouraged Steve to free associate and write on particular topics. A second used overlearned material from childhood, such as *The Three Bears*. Steve's task was to retell the story on paper for his son Scott. This gave him the support of a predetermined story, but still required that he impose structure on it in the retelling. When he could not remember a story, a cloze technique was used to aid recall. For example, the first prompt for *The Three Bears* was "Once upon a time there was a little girl with golden curls named..." As he progressed through a story, the clinician used fewer prompts, until a simple "and then..." was sufficient.

On one occasion Steve created a unique ending to this familiar story that helped him recognize and explore his feelings of rage and frustration over his helplessness. Instead of the usual ending where Goldilocks awakes to see the bears looking at her and immediately runs home, he wrote: [sic]

"The baby on the other hand saw someone in his bed. Papa Bear went growling after her and woke her up something terrible. From there on she was frightened as all get out. She then fainted. Papa

Bear then left her alone, he didn't know what else to do. What a confusing moment! After Papa and Mama Bears when down to eat, Golielocks woke up and beat baby bear then headed down stairs. Since she had just warmed up on baby bear, papa bear was no problem, not that Baby Bear was tough or anything, it was just the round of practice that was such a help. So she punched on Papa Bear for quite a while, until he got tired of it and collapsed. Mama Bear was so shoked and surprise that she just knelet down by Papa Bear and shut up. At that time Goldielocks just went on home. Papa Bear woke in a fit of range and didn't talk about it again after that night. The same went for Baby Bear. And Mama Bear didn't dare mention it to papa bear again after than night. So they all went about their quiet ways and kept their mouths shut. The end."

When questioned about his version of what happened to Papa Bear, Steve remarked with uncharacteristic fluent speech and a surprised look of recognition, "It's me, I didn't know I was writing about myself!"

Dysarthria. Steve continued to make improvements in voicing, breath control, and articulation. He used a watch that chimed every hour to remind him to do periodic voicing drills. Steve's speech intelligibility was significantly enhanced by structured treatment situations presented as language stimulation for his son who could not always understand him. This treatment was designed to allow them to interact in a relaxed context and to give Scott opportunities to learn his father's "dysarthric dialect." Several children's games were used to stimulate these interactions. In the first session Scott could not follow the simple directions Steve gave him and looked to his mother to interpret. For the first time Steve and Laura became aware that Scott was not being stubborn; he really could not understand his father. In later sessions Scott and Steve developed a remarkable patience with each other. On one occasion, when Steve was teaching Scott the names of musical instruments, Scott needed 10 repetitions before he could understand and repeat the name "accordian." The intense and loving attention each gave the other in these exercises formed a foundation for other father and son interactions that developed later.

Phase III: Independent Outpatient Period (13 to 25 MPO)

Therapeutic goals in this period focused on consolidating reacquired skills, using these skills independently, and developing ways to compensate for persisting communication and cognitive deficits. Two developments marked the beginning of this phase. First, Steve was loaned a computer system to use at home. Second, he began work as a volunteer at the Veterans Administration Medical Center. This activity required him to talk with persons who did not know him and were unfamiliar with his impairments.

Computer Based Treatment. Steve was now taught to use the computer to assist him in carrying out some activities of daily living. While he continued to use software that focused on the foundation skills of attention, memory, and reading, he also learned how to use the *Personal Finance Manager* software package to manage the family checkbook and budgeting. Because his wife had found this task frustrating, Steve's resumption of his previous role was very important.

With the help of the computer Steve was also able to assume some responsibilities as a father. This was important because it helped to restore a balance in his relationship with his son. Because of his decreased capacity to initiate speech, his spontaneous comments to his son were often reactive or negative. By using software designed for use in teaching a variety of concepts and skills to preschool children, he had a means of interacting with Scott that replaced what he could not implement on his own. Using the computer Steve has been able to communicate more successfully with his son. Each of them has been clearly delighted with the teaching and learning that they share while using the computer.

Finally, the computer became a vehicle for enhancing communication between Steve and Laura. Steve began keeping a journal with the computer. He used it to vent his feelings and to record things he needed to remember. Laura had often felt "cut off" from what Steve was experiencing because he could not communicate well in conversation. After he logged his ideas in his journal, however, she could read what concerned him and they had a basis for discussion. In this way the computer has become a counseling aid, giving support to each of them and providing a vehicle for resolution of their problems.

Summary of Steve's Case Study

Steve's case illustrates that the microcomputer has some useful applications and can provide unexpected benefits in the rehabilitation of the head-injured patient. Traditional microcomputer training applications have allowed him to work independently and to rebuild basic cognitive and communicative skills. Nontraditional microcomputer applications have permitted Steve to gain insight into his feelings about himself and allowed him to reasume some of his roles as father, husband, and household manager. Because it is not dedicated to any single function, the microcomputer will continue to have value as Steve's rehabilitation progresses and his needs change.

Steve remains dysarthric, but he is increasingly successful in talking with those who know him and with strangers who take time to listen. His position, a volunteer, which requires that he deliver charts and lab specimens within the medical center, has added to his sense of self-worth. His ability to book his own dial-a-ride transportation by telephone, his use of an electric wheelchair, and his walking with the use of a quad-cane have given him increased freedom. He demonstrates this increased freedom by riding his adult tricycle around the bike paths at a local park, accompanied by his son on a Big Wheel.

Steve continues to have difficulty in initiating, planning, organizing, evaluating priorities, and remembering. He remains generally slow in all physical and intellectual activity. However, he has a realistic awareness of what he has lost. He has experienced periods of depression, but his personal strengths appear to be undiminished by his injuries. These strengths include a buoyant sense of humor, an ability to persist despite repeated failure, and a charismatic sweetness of personality. Although it is difficult to know whether further progress will be made, it is clear that the microcomputer has significantly affected his recovery. At this time he senses that he can still make a contribution to society. Despite the coexistence of serious residual disabilities, this return of a sense of self-worth and a capacity for relating to others is a hallmark of successful rehabilitation.

POSTSCRIPT

Traditionally, clinicians have used computers to provide massed practice on a variety of tasks. This application was seen in the treatment of Chuck's aphasia. However, George Kelly, an eminent clinical psychologist, has pointed out that a person's experience is not measured by the number of events with which he collides, but by the investments he has made in the process. Chuck was a computer programmer and was able to feel some continuity with his past identity by working with the computer. Steve, however, was intrigued by the glamor of this new technology and impressed with its power to reveal his integrity to himself and others. Surely the positive feelings of each man in receiving portions of his treatment via computer must account for some degree of its success.

In some respects, it is easy for clinicians to see why the programmed learning presented to Chuck lent itself well to the microcomputer presentation. Its ability to control stimuli, time events, measure responses, and control treatment progression can greatly increase the clinician's capabilities. On the other hand, it is not easily seen that the same device can have psychosocial value as was seen in Steve's case. The true power of this technology seems to be that it can serve clinicians and patients in a multitude of ways, only a few of which we have yet conceived.

The case reports presented in this chapter support the inclusion of computerized therapy as one more tool in the clinician's arsenal. When selectively used by an informed and discriminating clinician, computerized treatment can yield positive results. But, it is important to realize that this technology is still limited. Much must be left to the clinician. Human communication remains an interpersonal experience and the clinician will remain the dominant member of the clinician-computer-patient rehabilitation team with the responsibility of determining when, in what ways, and with whom the technology should be used.

REFERENCES

Colarusso, R.P., & Hammill, D.D. (1972). *Motor Free Visual Perception Test*. Novato, CA: Academic Therapy Publications.

Dunn, Lloyd M., & Dunn, Leota M. (1981). *Peabody Picture Vocabulary Test–Revised* (PPVT-R). Circle Pines, MN: American Guidance Service.

Fitch, J.L., & Cross, S.T. (1983). Telecomputer treatment for aphasia. *Journal of Speech and Hearing Disorders, 48,* 335–336.

Goodglass, H., & Kaplan, E. (1972). *The assessment of aphasic and related disorders.* Philadelphia: Lea and Febiger.

LaPointe, L., Horner, J. (1979). *Reading Comprehension Battery for Aphasia.* Tigard, OR: C.C. Publications.

Porch, B.E. (1967). *Porch Index of Communicative Ability.* Palo Alto, CA: Consulting Psychologists Press.

Schuell, H.M. (1965). *Minnesota Test for Differential Diagnosis of Aphasia.* Minnesota: University of Minnesota Press.

Spreen, O., & Benton, A.L. (1969). *Neurosensory Center Comprehensive Examination for Aphasia.* Victoria, BC: Department of Psychology, University of Victoria.

Teasdale, G., & Jennett, B. (1974). Assessment of coma and impaired consciousness. *Lancet, 101,* 81–84.

APPENDIX A: Selected Software Used with Steve and Target Goals

Key:
1. Attention and reaction time
2. Memory
3. Reading comprehension
4. General information
* Steve used with his son

Alien Addition/Meteor Multiplication/Minus Mission (1,4)
(Developmental Learning Materials)

Analogies (3)
(Hartley Courseware)

Arithmetic Skills (4)
(Edu-ware)

Bank Street Writer (word processor)
(Broderbund)

Birth of a Phoenix (2,3)
(Phoenix)

Cloze Plus and Comprehension Power (2,3)
(Milliken)

Cog-Rehab (1,2)
(Life Science Associates)

Compu-read (1,2,3)
(Edu-ware)

Dragon's Keep (2,3)*
(Sierra on-line)

Elementry Vo. #7 (2)*
(Minnesota Educational Computer Consortium)

Facemaker (2)*
(Spinnaker Software)

Game Show/Tic-Tac-Show (3,4)
(Computer Advanced Ideas)

Micro Read (2,3)
(American Educational Computer, Inc.)

Murder by the Dozen (2,3)
(CBS Software)

Olympic Decathalon (1)
(Microsoft)

Perception (1,2)
(Edu-ware)

Preschool IQ Builder (1,4)*
(Program Design, Inc.)

SAT English I (3)
(Microlab Learning Center)

SAT (3,4)
(Harcourt, Brace, Jovanovich)

Sink the Ship (1)*
(User Contributed Software)

Understanding Sentences/Understanding Stories (2,3)
(Sunset Software)

Word Memory Program (1,3)
(Bell and Howell)

APPENDIX B: Steve's Word Processing Samples

Sample #1: OCTOBER 1983 - (Note Steve's expressed sense of loss and depression.)

[SIC]
LAURA HAS BEEN MY WIFE FOR OVER FOUR YEARS NOW, AND SHE IS THE GREATEST THING THAT HAS OCURRED TO ME IN MY LIFETIME. I DON'T THINK I CAME TO REALLY KNOW THAT UNTIL AFTER THE ACCIDENT, WHEN I BECAME A REAL CRIPPLE, A PERSON WHO DIDN'T KNOW UP FROM DOWN. THAT WAS WHEN I REALLY APPESIATED HER COMPANNY. NOW I HAVE ALL KINDS OF ROTTEN THOUGHTS RUNNING THROUGH MY HEAD, AND MOST OF THEM ARE NOT TO LOVELY, BUT LIKE JUST ABOUT EVERYTHING ELSE, IT IS IN ONE EARY AND OUT THE OTHER. AND SHE NEVER HEARS A WORD OF IT. JUST AS WELL!!! I CAN'T REMEMBER TOO MUCH FROM BEFORE WE WERE MARRIED AND EVEN BEFORE THAT, MY MEMORY ISN'T TOO GOOD. WELL HERE I AM AT THE TYPEWRITER AGAIN, WHAT A DUMMY! I SHOULD BE WRITTING THIS THING, AND ERASEING MY MISTAKES INSTEAD OF DELETING THEM.

Sample #2: FEBRUARY 1984 - (Note the general awkwardness of topic introduction and sentence construction in some sentences.)

[SIC]
DEAR MOM AND DAD,
  YESTERDAY, MONDAY, I VOLUNTEERED AS A DELIVERY-PERSON AND HAD A GREAT TIME. I WENT FROM 9:20 TO 4:15. I GOT THERE BY BUS, THEN I TRADED MY CHAIR FOR A MOTORIZED WHEELCHAIR - ONLY FOR THE DAY. ABOUT IN A MONTH I WILL HAVE MY OWN. ONLY MINE WILL BE SORT OF A CART WITH SWIVEL SEAT AND HANDLEBARS. NOW MOM, DON'T WORRY ABOUT THE MOTOR - IT HAS A HIGH AND LOW SPEED. I WILL KEEP IT ON LOW, YESTERDAY I DIDN'T GO INTO ``HIGH'' AT ALL. THE PURPOSE OF THE ELECTRIC WHEELCHAIR IS TO SPEED ME UP TO WHERE OTHER PEOPLE CAN WALK, AND KEEP THAT SPEED. THE LOW SPEED GOES 3 MPH, AND THE HIGH SPEED GOES 6 MPH.
  I GOT MORE SLEEP THAN USUAL AT YOUR HOUSE. I DON'T KNOW WHY, BUT I GOT OVER 8 HOURS OF SLEEP

COMPARED TO MY USUAL OF 6 HOURS EVERYWHERE ELSE.
 PAM SPOKE TO MY PHISICAL THERAPIST TODAY AND SHE SAID IT WOULD BE O.K. FOR ME TO COME IN ONCE A WEEK TO WORK OUT A BIT. THAT IS GREAT! THE REASON SHE HADN'T SET UP MY SCHEDULE BEFORE IS BECAUSE SHE WANTED TO WORK AROUND MY VOLUNTEER SCHEDUAL. I DIDN'T HAVE THAT COMPLETED YET AND I STILL DON'T. I WANT TO FIND OUT WHAT IS BEST FOR ME. MAYBE GETTING AS MUCH TIME IN AS POSSIBLE WOULD HELP ME IN THE LONG RUN, I AM NOT SURE YET. WELL I WILL STOP FOR NOW, AND START IT UP IN A FEW WEEKS - THE LETTER IS WHAT I WILL START UP AGAIN.
                             LOVE,

Sample #3: APRIL 1984 - (Free association about his son, Scott: Note Steve's partially intact capacity to think abstractly about his relationships.)

[SIC]
 I THINK I SHOULD BE A LITTLE MORE A PART OF HIS LIFE. NOT JUST HIS FATHER, BUT MORE LIKE A FRIEND. WELL WHAT I MEAN BY THAT IS I SHOULD BE SOMEONE HE CAN TALK TO ABOUT WHAT HE EXPECTS AND DOESN'T EXPECT, WHAT HE WOULD IGNORE, AND WHAT HE EXPECTS AND DOESNT EXPECT FROM HIS MOTHER AND FATHER. THAT WOULD REALLY BE HELPFUL. SCOTT SHOULD BE A REALL CHALLENGE BECAUSE OF HIS SMART PUSCH AS A YOUNG MAN AND HIS QUESTIONING LITTLE MIND. HIS MIND ISN'T SO LITTLE THESE DAYS. HE IS PRETTY DARN INTELLIGENT LITTLE CUSS FOR SUCH A YOUNG MAN, AND A YOUNG MAN HE IS. I AM SO PROUD OF HIM.

AUTHOR INDEX

Ahern, M.B., 20
Aronson, A.F., 145
Aten, James L., 1, 3, 7, 8–9, 10, 15, 60, 119–131, 168
Baer, D.M., 15, 226
Barresi, B., 2
Barrett, M., 190
Baskey, P., 168
Basso, A., 1, 7, 60
Benson, D.F., 37
Benton, A.L., 62, 78, 121, 145, 247
Beukelman, D., 147
Bierwisch, M., 146
Boning, R., 191, 220, 222
Borkowski, J.G., 62
Bressler, E., 190
Brink, J., 147
Broca, Paul, 2
Broida, H., 1, 7, 60
Brookshire, R.H., 2, 33, 200, 205, 218
Brown, J.P., 145
Brubaker, S., 36, 190
Brutten, E., 25
Buck, M., 37
Buckingham, H.W., 146
Butfield, E., 60
Caligiuri, M.P., 1, 7, 60, 130, 168
Callahan, S., 93
Canter, G.J., 146
Capitani, E., 1, 60
Chapey, R., 1, 3, 4, 12–13, 86, 183–195, 221, 241
Chwat, S., 45
Cicone, M., 168
Colarusso, R.P., 255
Collins, Michael J., 3, 8–9, 10, 105–118, 61, 146, 171
Conway, William F., 3, 10–11, 151–166
Cousins, N., 23

Custer, D.D., 38
Dans, J., 45
Darley, F.L., 1, 145, 147, 201
Datta, K.D., 60
Davis, A.G., 1, 2, 13, 14, 35–36, 116–117, 168, 189, 226, 241
Davis, G.A., 45, 90
Deal, J.L., 60, 61, 93
Deal, L.A., 60, 93
DeRenzi, E., 33, 62, 199
Dodaro, R., 87
Dunn, Leota M., 199, 255
Dunn, Lloyd M., 199, 255
Dwyer, C., 61
Eisenson, J., 2, 69
Feyerson, P.S.X., 147
Fioldi, N., 168
Fitzpatrick, P.M., 2
Florance, Cheri L., 3, 10–11, 151–166
Fokes, F.J., 230
Freese, Arthur, 37
Friden, T., 61
Gardner, H., 168
Garland, G., 45
Gaughan, M., 87
Geschwind, N., 145, 146
Goldstein, K., 186
Golper, L., 168
Goodglass, H., 8, 21, 78–80, 110, 121, 143, 186, 199, 255
Grossman, R., 145
Guilford, J.P., 184, 186, 187
Gurland, G., 45
Hagen, C., 1, 147
Hammill, D.D., 255
Harris, E.H., 20
Hart, H.S., 226, 227
Helm, N., 146, 149
Helm-Estabrooks, N.A., 2, 171

Author Index

Hoepfner, R., 186, 187
Hoffer, Pamela C., 4, 15, 16, 245–266
Holland, A.L., 1, 7, 60, 121, 127, 130, 147, 168, 223, 226
Holloran, S., 190
Horner, J., 78, 121, 221, 248, 255
Huisingh, R., 190
Jenkins, J.J., 5, 29
Jennett, B., 254
Jiminez-Pabon, E., 5, 29
Jorgensen, C., 190
Kaplan, E., 8, 21, 78–80, 110, 121, 143, 186, 199, 255
Kearns, K.P., 3–4, 14, 15, 219, 225–244
Keith, R.L., 38
Kelly, George, 262
Kertesz, A., 1
Kilpatrick, K., 190
Kitselman, K., 61
Knox, A., 188
Kubler-Ross, E.K., 188
Kushner, H., 188

LaPointe, L.L., 14, 61, 66, 68, 78, 121, 128, 220, 221, 248, 255
Lazzari, A., 190
Lemme, M.L., 20
Lemmer, E., 87
Levin, H., 145, 146
Levita, E., 168
Lezak, M.D., 203
Lieberman, A., 37
Liles, B.Z., 205
Lincoln, N.B., 60
Linebaugh, C., 45
Loverso, F.L., 13–14, 89, 98, 219
Lubinski, R., 3, 10, 11–12, 112, 167–181, 187
Luria, A.R., 146
Manchester, R.B., 36
Marshall, R.C., 1–16, 197–213, 60, 61, 168, 193
Martin, A.D., 13, 35, 184, 212
Martin, A.I., 146, 147
McCrae-Cochrane, R., 241
McNeil, M.R., 221
McReynolds, L.V., 231, 242
Mills, R.H., 4, 15, 16, 245–266

Milton, S.B., 241
Minifie, F., 16
Morh, J., 108, 146, 147
Morganstein, S., 190
Morrison, E., 168, 187
Moss, C.S., 37
Neisser, U., 184
Newhoff, M., 45
Parker, W., 147
Peters, P., 190
Pettit, J.M., 168
Philips, L., 168
Phillips, D.S., 1, 60, 160
Pickersgill, M.J., 60
Plum, F., 145
Porch, B.E., 7, 34, 49, 61, 62, 77, 90, 92, 93, 110, 112, 121, 134, 145, 157, 186, 199, 217, 218, 221, 227, 247
Porec, J., 7, 145
Posner, J., 145
Prescott, Thomas E., 215–225, 3, 12, 13, 14, 89, 98
Rau, Marie T., 3, 4, 5, 6, 13, 31–44, 168
Raven, J.C., 62, 110, 121
Rigrodsky, S., 168, 187
Risley, T.R., 226
Rosenbek, J.C., 3, 19, 20, 23, 61, 68, 146
Sanders, P., 45
Sanders, S.B., 3, 7, 8, 89–104
Sands, E., 60, 168
Sarno, M.T., 60, 168
Scheerer, E., 186
Schuell, H., 5, 29, 33, 60–61, 171, 186, 199, 247
Searle, J.R., 212
Selinger, J., 13–14, 89, 98
Selinger, M., 219
Shankweiler, D., 60
Shewan, C.M., 1
Shoemaker, D., 25
Silverman, M., 60, 168
Skelly, M., 136, 146, 228
Sklar, M., 20
Smith, A., 7, 60
Smith, M., 190
Sneeden, M., 190
Sparks, R., 2, 127
Spreen, O., 62, 78, 121, 247

Stokes, T.F., 15, 226
Teasdale, G., 254
Thompson, C.K., 14, 219
Tompkins, C.A., 1, 60, 168
Towey, M.P., 168
VanDemark, A.A., 78–88, 3, 7, 8
Vignolo, L.A., 1, 33, 60, 62, 199
Vogel, Deanie, 3, 4, 5, 6, 19–29
Warren, R.L., 133–149, 3, 4, 8–9, 10, 60
Webster, E.J., 45–58, 3, 6
Wechsler, D., 49, 159
Weigl, E., 146
Wepman, J.M., 13, 19, 35, 36, 60, 184–185, 189, 212
Wertz, R.T., 1, 3, 4, 7, 8, 20, 38, 59–73, 42, 60, 61, 68, 93, 131, 146
Wilcox, M.J., 2, 13, 35–36, 116–117, 168, 189, 226, 241
Wilson, Robert, 32–44
Wolpe, J., 25
Wulf, H.H., 37
Yorkston, D., 147
Young, Charles H., 45

Zachman, L., 190
Zangwill, O., 60

SUBJECT INDEX

Accountability, 17
Activities of Daily Living (ADL), 160, 163
Acute care hospital, 33
Adult Communication Analysis, 157
Akinetic mutism, 145
Alien Addition (computer program), 258
Ambivalence, 49–50
Ameri-Ind Gestural Code, 136
Amnesia, 255
Analysis of Interaction Dynamics, 157
Anger, 50–51
Anomic aphasia, 199
Antidepressant drugs, 165
Apraxia
   automatic speech in, 127
   in Broca's aphasia, 229
   communicative status in, 125–126, 129
   continuancy training in, 127–129
   limb, 146
   minimizing struggle in, 205–206
   performance disparities in, 129–130
   performance stability in, 123
   severs, 9
   in severe aphasia, 48
   speech evaluation in, 122–123, 129
   in stroke, 94, 120, 201
   treatment of
      measuring effects of, 130
      self-assisted, 126
      traditional, 121–126
Articulation, 136
Ataxic aphasia. *See* Broca's aphasia
Auditory comprehension. *See* Comprehension
Augmentative communication, 9, 10, 137–138, 147–148
Automatic speech, 127
Bank Street Writer (word-processor), 258

Base 10 Response Forms, 66, 68
Baseline data, 15
Behavior
   change, 159
   jcompensatory, 201–204
   refocusing of, 204–205
Bibliotherapy, 37
Boston Diagnostic Aphasia Examination (BDAE)
   in apraxia, 1212, 123–125, 130
   in chronic aphasia, 7–8, 78–84
   in cognitive treatment, 186, 193
   computer-administered, 255
   in global aphasia, 110
   in head injury, 143
   in high level aphasia, 21
   in reading deficits, 200–201
   in stroke, 199
Broca's aphasia, 9, 106, 199
   in head injury, 134, 145
   speech evaluation in, 21–23
   verbal elaboration in
      clinical probes, 232
      continued treatment rationale, 229–230
      defined, 233–234
      experimental design, 231–235
      generalization in, 238–239
      mataerials for, 230–231
      patient description in, 227–228
      purpose of, 227
      response definition in, 232
      response elaboration training, 227
      response scoring, 232
      results of, 235–242
      scoring reliability in, 235
      test results in, 235–240
      treatment goal, 230
      treatment history, 228–229
      treatment phase, 232–235

See also Global aphasia
Center for Independent Living, 11, 151–166
Cerebrovascular accident. *See* Stroke
Chronic aphasia
   speech evaluation in, 62–65
   treatment of, 6–8, 65–66
Clinical Aphaseology Conference, 14
Clinical data, 14
Clinical probes, 232
Clinician
   client and, 2–3
   computer vs., 15–16
   flexibility of, 12–14
   in nursing home, 179
   rehabilitative role of, 28
Cognition
   problem-solving and, 158–161
   role of, 11
Cognitive approach
   counseling in, 188–189
   medical history in, 185
   results of, 192–194
   social history in, 185–186
   speech evaluation in, 186–188
   treatment, 188–192
Cog Rehab Program (computer program), 257
Coloured Progressive Matrices, 62, 110, 121
Communication
   in apraxia, 125–126, 129
   augmentative, 137–138
   in global aphasia, 114–117
   in head injury, 136–148
   in stroke, 157, 160
   as treatment goal, 15
   See also Social communication
Communication Activities in Daily Living, 123–125, 130, 168, 223
Compensatory behaviors, 201–204
Compliance, 160
Comprehension
   auditory
     in apraxia, 121–122
     in Broca's aphasia, 229
     in global aphasia, 116, 248–249
     heightening of, 205
   microcomputers in, 251–252, 255–256
   in stroke, 93, 94
   cognitive approach to, 186
   reading
     in apraxia, 122
     deficits in, 200–202
     microcomputers in, 249–254
     in stroke, 95–96, 108
Compu-Read (computer program), 258
Computers. *See* Microcomputers
Concentration/denial, 158
Conduction aphasia, 199
Continuancy training, 127–129
Controlling struggle, 23–24
Convergent production, 187, 191
Convergent thinking, 184, 221–222
Conversation
   cognitive approach to, 187–188
   in high level aphasia, 24–25
Coping, 158–160
Coping and Compliance Assessment, 158
Counseling, 4–5
   cognitive approach to, 188–189
   family, 203
   in high level aphasia, 37–42
   spouse, 96
   in stroke, 203
Data
   baseline, 15
   clinical, 14
Defense mechanisms, 158
Delay, in word retrieval, 207
Denial/concentration, 158
Dependent outpatient treatment, 258–260
Depression, 165
Description, 207
Dictation, 24
Discourse, 187–188
Divergent production, 187, 191–192
Divergent thinking, 184, 221–222
Drawing, 115–116
Drug therapy, 165
Dysarthria, 260
Dysgraphia, 201
Evaluation. *See* Speech, evaluation of
Evaluative thinking, 184, 187, 192

Subject Index 273

Examining for Aphasia, 69
Experimental design, 231–235
Expressive aphasia. *See* Broca's aphasia
Facilitation, 146–147
Family
 counseling of, 6
 dynamics of, 202–203
 See also Spousal role
Family Administered Home Assessment, 155
Family Interaction Analysis, 157, 161
Fibrillation, 159
Financial management, 155
Flexibility, 12–14
Follow-up
 in global aphasia, 117–118
 in head injury, 142–143
 in high level aphasia, 28–, 40–42
 in stroke, 209–210
Function Recognition (computer program), 249
Game Show (computer program), 251, 253
Gelb-Goldstein-Weigl-Scheerer Object Scoring Test, 186
Generalization, 207, 238–239
Gesturing
 in Broca's aphasia, 229
 in global aphasia, 114–115
 in head injury, 136
 in stroke, 94
Getting the Main Ideas and Using the Context, 220
Glasgow Coma Scale, 254–255
Global aphasia, 9
 auditory comprehension in, 116
 communication aids in, 114–117
 follow-up, 117–118
 initial observation, 106–107
 prognosis in, 107–108
 speech evaluation in, 108, 116
 total communication in, 114–117
 treatment of
  early, 108–109
  formal, 110
  patient's response to, 113–114
  planning of, 110–113
  results of, 117

 See also Broca's aphasia
Goals
 clinician, 23–28
 patient
  in chronic aphasia, 8, 28
  in high level aphasia, 23, 25, 34–35, 39
Graphic skills, 95
Group treatment, 96
Guilford Structure of Intellect Model, 184
Handi-Voice, 9, 133, 138, 143, 147
Head injuries
 augmentative communication in, 137–141, 147–148
 final outcome in, 143–145
 follow-up in, 142–145
 initial evaluation of, 134–135
 return of speech after, 141–147
 speech disorder in, 145–148
 total communication in, 136–137
Hemiplegia, 48–49, 153–154, 227, 228
High level aphasia
 clinician goals in, 23–28
 controlling struggle in, 23–24
 conversational practice in, 24–25
 counseling in, 37–42
 early intervention in, 20–21
 follow-up in, 28–29, 40–42
 medical history in, 32–33
 patient goals in, 23, 25
 return to work after, 39–42
 speaking hierarchy in, 25–28
 speech evaluation in, 21–23, 33–34
 treatment stages in, 34–42
Histories. *See* Medical history; Social history
Home safety, 156
Homes, nursing. *See* Nursing homes
Hypertension, 198, 216
Imitation, 234
The Independent Living Self-Assessment, 155
Independent outpatient treatment, 260–261
Indirect therapy, 35
Inpatient treatment, 257–258
Institutionalized clients, 11–12

Subject Index

Intellectual ability, 158–159
Intensive treatment. *See* Treatment, residential
Isolatio/objectivity, 158
Jacksonian seizure, 25
Judgment, of patient, 5–6
Laboratory findings, in stroke, 154
Language and thought, 12–13
Langauge Master, 66, 116
Limb apraxia, 146
Linguistic structure, 15
Listener "fill-in", 27
Listening, 107
Logical analysis/rationalization, 158
Mammoth Book of Word Games, 36
Meal planning, 156
Medical history
  in cognitive treatment, 185
  geriatric, 153–154
  in high level aphasia, 32–33
  in residential treatment, 76
  in stroke evaluation, 153–154, 198, 216
Melodic Intonation Therapy, 1–2, 127
Memory
  cognitive approach to, 187, 191, 193
  defects of, 255
  defined, 184
Memowriter, 55, 56
Memphis State University Speech and Hearing Clinic, 6
Memphis Veterans Administration Medical Center, 90–91
Mental disease, 158
Meteor Multiplication (computer program), 258
Microcomputers
  as communication tool, 261
  in dysarthria treatment, 260
  non-traditional application of, 16
  in speech evaluation, 247–248, 255–256
  task selection by, 248–251
  treatment with, 15–16
    dependent outpatient, 258–260
    independent outpatient, 260–261
    inpatient, 257–258
Micro Read (computer program), 258

Minnesota Test for Differential Diagnosis of Aphasia
  in chronic aphasia, 60–61
  in cognitive treatment, 186, 193
  in global aphasia, 247
  institutional application of, 171, 178
  in reading deficits, 200–201, 253
  in stroke, 199
Minus Mission (computer program), 258
Motor aphasia. *See* Broca's aphasia
Motor Free Visual Perception Test, 255
Motor programming, 147
Multiple baseline study, 15
Mutism, 9–10, 145
Nonfluent aphasia. *See* Broca's aphasia
Nursing homes
  clinician changes in, 179
  environment of, 168, 172–173
Objectivity/isolation, 158
Object Sorting Test, 186
Occupational therapy, 155–156, 160, 163–165
Oral nonverbal apraxia, 110
Oral-Verbal Apraxia Battery, 157
Outpatient treatment
  computerized, 258–261
  in stroke, 211–212
PACE. *See* "Promoting Aphasics' Communicativeness Effectiveness"
Patients
  aphasia's impact on, 5
  clinician's relationship with, 2–3
  defined, 2
  elderly, 153–154
  goals of, 28
  high level clients, 5
  institutionalized, 11–12
  judgment of, 5–6
  listener reactions and, 28
  status appraisal, 159–161
Peabody Picture Vocabulary Test, 199, 201, 255
Performance, in apraxia, 123, 129–130
Personal Finance Manager (computer program), 261
Pharmacological interventions, 165
Phonation, 136
Phonetic assocation, 207

Physical examination, 154
Porch Index of Communicative Ability
  in cognitive treatment, 186, 193
  computerized use of, 254
  conditions used in
    apraxia, 121–125, 130, 208–209
    Broca's aphasia, 227, 228, 240
    chronic aphasia, 7–8, 62–68, 79–83
    global aphasia, 110–113, 247
    head injuries, 134, 140–145
    hemiplegia, 227, 228
    high level aphasia, 34, 38
    senescence, 152
    severe aphasia, 48–49
    stroke, 48–49, 53, 55, 57, 92–93, 97, 121, 157, 199, 210–212, 217–220, 222
  in evaluating treatment, 14, 15
  institutional application of, 77, 78
  in terminating treatment, 90–91
Portland Veterans Administration Medical Center, 33–34
Preposition Recognition (computer program), 249, 252
Preschool I.Q. Builder (computer program), 250
Probes, treatment, 98–103
Programming
  motor, 147
  sentence, 139–141
"Promoting Aphasics' Communicative Effectiveness" (PACE), 2, 13, 189
  in Broca's aphasia, 241
  in global aphasia, 116–117
Prostatic cancer, 222
Psychiatric disease, 158

Rationalization/logical analysis, 158
Eeact (computer program), 257
Reading comprehension. *See* Comprehension
Reading Comprehension Battery for Aphasis, 78, 83, 84, 121, 123–125, 130, 221, 247–248, 255
Recovery
  determination of, 90–91
  group treatment in, 96
  individual treatment in, 94–95
  reading comprehension in, 95–96
  speech evaluation in, 92–93
  verbing programs in, 98–103
Reentering treatment, 220–223
Refocusing behavior, 204–205
Rehabilitation
  clinician's role in, 28
  vocational, 137–138
Residential Aphasia Clinic (University of Michigan), 7, 75–88
Residential treatment
  evaluation data in, 78–80
  intensive, 77–78
  medical history in, 76
  outpatient, 77
  significant others in, 10–15
Responses
  definition of, 232
  elaboration training in, 227
  latency of, 252
  of patients, 112–114
Retention deficits, 200–201
Return of speech, 141–145
Return to work, 39–40
Revised Token Test, 221
Role changes, 12

SAT (computer program), 258
SAT English (computer program), 258
Scientific inquiry, 14–16
Scoring reliability, 235
Self-care, 155
Self-cueing strategies, 186
Sense of well-being, 158
Sentence programming, 139–141
Severe aphasia. *See* Global aphasia
Sharp Memowriter, 55, 56
Shell Games (computer program), 250
Shopping, 156
Significant others, 10–15, 169–170
Sink the Ship (computer program), 257
Sklar Aphasia Scale, 20
Social communication
  environment of, 168, 172–173
  goals of, 173
  observations in, 171–172
  problems of, 179–180
  speech evaluation in, 171
  strategies of, 173–177
  treatment outcomes in, 178–180

treatment strategies in, 173–177
underlying assumptions of, 169–170
Social history, 185–186
Spastic dysarthria, 260
Speaking situations, 25–28
Specific Skill Series, 220, 222
Speech
  automatic, 127
  deficits, management of, 8–10
  evaluation of
    cognitive approach to, 186–188
    computer applications, 250
    in defining maximum recovery, 92–93
    in elderly persons, 11
    in residential treatment, 78–80
    social communications approach to, 171
  importance of, 10
  inability to understand, 27
  return of, 141–145
  thought stimulation in, 12–13
  See also specific speech disorders
Spousal role
  ambivalence of, 49–50
  anger in, 50–51
  changing relationship, 55–57
  counseling, 96
  overprotection in, 52
Square Pairs (computer program), 250, 253
Stimuli, verbing, 99–103, 244
Stroke
  accepting limitations after, 43
  behavior after, 159, 203–205
  cognitive effects, 159
  comprehension deficits after, 93, 94, 200–202
  coping in, 158–159
  counseling in, 203–204
  drug therapy in, 165
  financial management in, 155
  follow-up in, 209–210
  individual treatment of, 94–95
  laboratory findings in, 154
  medical history in, 153–154, 198, 216
  occupational therapy in, 155–156, 161–163

outpatient treatment of, 211–212
patient status appraisal in, 159–161
physical examination in, 154
re-entering treatment for, 200–203
retention deficits after, 200–201
self-care in, 155
speech evaluation in, 92–93, 161–163, 198–202, 210–211, 216–218
support systems in, 155
termination of treatment after, 95–96
transportation evaluation after, 156
See also Apraxia
Stroke: The New Hope and the New Help, 37
Support systems, 155
Tactile naming, 146
Task selection, 248–251
Termination of treatment, 95–96
Theory, 4
Thinking
  convergent/divergent, 221–222
  evaluative, 184, 187, 192
Thought-centered therapy, 12–13, 35
Tic Tac Show (computer program), 251, 253
Token Test
  in apraxia, 121, 123–155
  in chronic aphasia, 62, 68, 78–84
  in global aphasia, 247
  in high level aphasia, 33, 38
  in retention deficits, 200, 201
  in stroke, 199
Training
  continuancy, 127–129
  vocational, 138–139
Transportation evaluation, 156
Treatment
  accountability in, 17
  advisability of, 7–8
  baseline data in, 15
  communication vs. linguistic form of, 15
  designs of, 14–15
  group, 96
  intensity of, 7–8
  outpatient, 211–212
  probes of, 98–103
  reentering, 220–223

scientific inquiry and, 14–16
significant others in, 10–15
termination of, 95–96
See also Outpatient treatment; Residential treatment; Social communications approach

Understanding Sentences (computer program), 258
Understanding Stories (computer program), 258
University of Michigan Residential Aphasia Clinic, 7, 75–88
Verbal apraxia, 229
Verbal communication. *See* Speech
Verbal elaboration training. *See* Broca's aphasia
Verbal program, 98–219
Veterans Administration Cooperative Study on Aphasia, 60
Visual Action Therapy, 2
Vocabulary training, 138–139
Vocational rehabilitation, 137–138
Wechsler Adult Intelligence Scale, 49, 159
Wernicke's aphasia, 106, 199
Word Fluency Measure, 62–68
Word processors, 258
Word Recognition Programs (computer programs), 249
Word retrieval, 94–95, 201, 206–208
Workbook for Aphasia, 36
Work, return to, 39–40
Writing
  in apraxia, 122
  computer testing of, 256
  to dictation, 24
  in global aphasia, 108, 116
  after stroke, 206